CHRIS WALKER

Keep The Weight Off

How To Naturally Control Your Weight For Life

I would like to dedicate this book to my little munchkin Donna whose encouragement, support and putting up with me writing this book means the whole world! I love you always.

Contents

Preface — ii

Why You Can't Keep The Weight Off — vi

She Hated Looking At Herself — 1

How To Stop Making Excuses — 8

Creating The New And Improved You — 16

Emotional Eating And That Big Jerk — 23

Modifying Your Emotional Blueprint — 32

Why You Shouldn't Surrender — 45

How To Eat Natural Foods — 55

10 Day Fresh Start Juice Fast — 66

Don't Make This Exercise Mistake — 73

Living Your New Healthy Life — 83

A Message From Your Body — 91

Chris's Motivational Quotes — 93

Praise From Clients — 101

Personal Support — 106

About the Author — 108

Preface

Why I Wrote This

Congratulations, ladies! You've taken the first step towards reclaiming your health and shedding those unwanted pounds. I'm here to equip you with some simple yet effective tools that will supercharge your weight loss journey. You see, I believe in you and your good intentions, but it's time to tackle the obstacles that have been standing in your way.

I wrote this for you because I wanted to empower you to make a change in the area of your health, in particular, your unwanted weight. I would like to share with you some very simple and effective tools that will help you to implement those good intentions of yours. Yes, I know you mean well and that you don't wish your body any intentional harm but something is getting in the way of your desired results and I would like to tell you what it is. In fact, I'm confident that If you follow my advice in this book you can finally get the weight loss results you're after and naturally control your weight for the rest of your life! Strong words, I know, but change is possible for you!

This book will dive deep into the powerful connection between your mind and body. We'll explore what I like to call your Emotional Blueprint and how it affects your weight loss efforts. No more emotional eating, bingeing, or stress-induced snacking! We're going to revamp your mindset and say goodbye to those negative behaviors that sabotage your goals.

Keeping the weight off has more to do with the mind-body connection than anything else. As we get into this book I'll be discussing your Emotional Blueprint and what needs to change about that so we can put an end to your emotional eating, fear of failure or any other negative behaviour contrary to your weight loss goals. Your Emotional Blueprint works in conjunction with your mind to give you a supportive mindset or what I call a Healthy Mindset. You cannot lose weight if you have unresolved emotional issues feeding into an Overweight Mindset. I really need you to get this because too many women think all they need to do is power through workouts, above all else and count calories to lose weight but nothing could be further from the truth. You can't lose emotional weight with diet and exercise alone.

Now, don't get me wrong. Eating a wholesome, natural diet and staying active is essential. You'll find plenty of tips on nutrition and exercise here. But here's the secret sauce: we can't ignore the emotional side of the equation. It's a neglected area of weight loss, but trust me, it's the key to lasting success.

I'm about to share with you diet and nutrition tips yes, but more importantly, what kind of mindset you need in order to lose your unwanted weight. I also want to identify any unsupportive behaviours or emotional hang-ups that you must correct if you want to lose weight permanently, in other words, keep it off!

Throughout this book, we'll talk about two mindsets that can make or break your journey. Let's meet them:

The Healthy Mindset

A healthy, slim, athletic build that some may refer to as a "toned" or "hard body". This person thinks positively about health and enjoys doing things to support his or her physique, like eating healthy foods and exercising. Self-love is at an all-time high and they often motivate others with their actions.

The Overweight Mindset

An unhealthy, overweight build that some may refer to as fat or obese. This person thinks negatively about health and struggles doing things to support a healthy physique, like eating healthy foods and exercise Self-love is a work in progress, and their actions may unintentionally demotivate others.

Please keep these definitions in mind as I will be referring to them often. Okay, let's begin!

What Makes Me An Expert?

But wait, who am I to guide you on this journey? Allow me to introduce myself. I'm your trusty companion—a former Personal Trainer, Holistic Nutritionist, Functional Diagnostic Nutrition Practitioner (that's a mouthful, I know!), and Weight Loss Coach. I've also incorporated techniques like Emotional

Freedom Technique (EFT), Neuro-Linguistic Programming (NLP), and Hypnosis, into my arsenal of tools.

My passion for health and fitness ignited when I tragically lost both my parents to illness. First my father from a stroke and complications in the hospital and then my mother to diabetes, and colon cancer. It drove me to learn everything I could about reclaiming health and overcoming weight struggles. Over the years, I've become a weight loss problem solver, specializing in helping women overcome emotional barriers, cleanse their bodies, and achieve optimal well-being. And let me tell you, emotional issues are often the real culprits behind weight loss roadblocks.

With over 18 years of experience and having helped thousands of women achieve their weight loss goals, I've learned a thing or two. I've witnessed patterns, mistakes, and victories. And guess what? The most significant factor that separates success from failure is none other than a Healthy Mindset! Forget the fad diets, the calorie counting, and the fitness gimmicks. It's time to transform your mindset and unlock the real secret to weight loss.

So, are you ready to buckle up and embark on this journey? Are you eager to discover new tools that will finally free you from stubborn fat? Get ready to say goodbye to cravings and overeating. It's time to unleash the best version of yourself! Let's jump right in and kick some weight-loss butt—metaphorically, of course!

Why You Can't Keep The Weight Off

Introduction

Alright, let's get real ladies. Before we dive into the nitty-gritty of weight loss, let's take a moment to see if this book is the right fit for you. I want to highlight some unsupportive behaviors that might resonate with you. If you find yourself nodding along to any of these, then we've got some work to do. So, here we go:

The "I Don't Deserve to Be Thin" Syndrome:

Deep down, you may feel like you don't deserve a healthy body. As a result, you haven't even mustered the courage to embark on your weight loss journey. But hey, let's kick that negative thinking to the curb, shall we?

The "Never Enough" Mindset:

You constantly doubt yourself, feeling like you're not smart, pretty, or good enough to have the body you desire. It's time to silence that inner critic and embrace your worthiness.

The Punishing Exercise Routine:

Exercise becomes a form of punishment for not losing weight, so you believe that more exercise is the answer. But trust me, there's a healthier and more balanced approach we'll explore together.

The Excuse Factory:

You find yourself using excuses like lack of money or time to avoid pursuing weight loss opportunities that deep down you know are good for you. It's time to break free from those limiting beliefs.

The Fear Monger:

Fear has become your constant companion, overshadowing the potential positive outcomes of improving your health and weight. We'll tackle those fears head-on and shift your focus to the incredible rewards awaiting you.

The Resentful Gaze:

You might feel a twinge of resentment toward healthy and fit individuals, even if you don't mean to. Don't worry, it happens, but we'll work on reshaping your perspective and fostering a supportive mindset.

The Belief Blockade:

You don't even believe that weight loss is possible for you, so you don't bother trying. It's time to ignite that spark of belief and prove your doubting self wrong.

The "Glass Half Empty" Syndrome:

You tend to focus on what's lacking in your life rather than what you truly desire. It's time to shift your perspective and embrace a more optimistic outlook.

The Underestimator:

You underestimate your true potential and what you can accomplish when you wholeheartedly focus on your health and weight. Get ready to unleash your hidden powers!

The Fear of Failure:

You let the fear of failure hinder you from seizing big opportunities that could lead to positive transformations. But guess what? Failure is just a stepping stone on the path to success, and we'll conquer that fear together.

Phew! That was quite a list. But here's the good news: all these self-sabotaging behaviors and false beliefs are fixable! Yes, you read that right. You have the power to change them, and I'm here to guide you through the process.

Please understand that this is all coming from a loving place and is just my observations of what I've come to understand about people over the years. If some or all of these things are going on inside of you, there's no wonder why you can't lose weight! All these things are enough to cripple anybody's weight loss efforts. I didn't even talk about diet and exercise yet, the stuff that people focus on the most, especially exercise.

Can you see how much internal conflict people are experiencing these days? The gyms are proof. So many women faithfully attend their gym, take fitness classes, bootcamps, hire personal trainers, and nutritionists, and still, they're not losing weight! Why? Because all of this emotional and mindset stuff is causing problems! Problems that need to be dealt with if you want to lose weight!

I've discovered this through my own healing journey after losing both my parents, by working on my own self-development, by keen observation, and by immersing myself in various disciplines like EFT (meridian psychotherapy), NLP, CBT, and neuroscience, I've uncovered strategies that can help you make lasting changes. But first, we need to address these internal conflicts that have been holding you back.

You see, all the focus on diets and exercise won't get you far if your subconscious mind is still playing a different tune. Your results are dictated by your subconscious beliefs, not the latest trendy diet or exercise routine. So, it's time to dig deep and bring those beliefs to light.

Awareness is key. You can't change what you're not aware of, my friend. And guess what else? Unhealed emotional wounds can wreak havoc on your health and prevent weight loss. So, if you've been scratching your head, wondering why the pounds won't budge despite your efforts, it's time to uncover the truth. It's your emotions and mindset that have been holding you hostage.

But fear not! We're here to tackle these challenges head-on. We'll focus on what truly matters first—your emotional well-being and mindset—and then we'll fine-tune your diet and fitness plan. Sound like a deal? Let's embark on this transformative journey together, shall we? It's time to rewrite your story and reclaim the body and health you deserve. Buckle up, my friend, we're in for an incredible ride!

She Hated Looking At Herself

My Keen Observation

"Ugggg!" she exclaimed, as she walked past the mirror, grunting disapprovingly. I leaned in, pretending I couldn't hear her, just to see what she would say. And then, she confessed with a sigh, "I absolutely hate looking at myself in the mirror." We both chuckled so it didn't become an awkward situation but I did make a mental note of it. Little did I know, this wasn't just an occasional thing. Nope, as a former personal trainer, I've seen this love-hate relationship play out time and time again with people trying to lose weight.

Now, don't get me wrong, there were a few guys who felt the same way. But let me tell you, the ladies took the cake when it came to this behavior. They were also as fickle as a feather in the wind, delicate as a porcelain teacup, and as fragile as a snowflake. The tiniest disappointment could send them spiraling. If they ate one wrong thing or didn't lose a pound that week, they would disappear for a while. Sure, they'd come up with some excuse for their absence, but eventually, they would just give up altogether!

After more than 10 years of observing the behaviors of weight loss seekers, I've learned a thing or two. And today, I'm going to share some of those lessons with you. These nuggets of wisdom might just help you out when you feel stuck in your weight loss journey or when you find yourself doing dumb things that go against your goals (we've all been there). So, without further ado, here are the valuable lessons I've learned from my experiences.

Lesson Number 1: Focus On What You Want

If you don't like looking at yourself in the mirror you're suggesting you hate yourself at present. Even deeper, you're focusing on what you do not like about yourself, and what you focus on expands, no pun intended. Ha, ha. In other words, It's essential to shift your focus from what you don't like about yourself to what you truly desire. When you constantly dwell on your flaws or imperfections, you attract more reasons and situations to stay the same.

Instead, practice self-love and acceptance in the present moment. Visualize the body, health, and fitness level you desire, and direct your attention toward the positive changes you want to manifest. You must first love yourself, be a peace with your present, then make plans for your future by focusing on what you do want. The body you want, the health you want, the fitness level you want, not what you don't want.

Lesson Number 2: Embrace The Power To Change

Don't be so caught up with what you see currently, rather realize you have the power and the ability to change. Once you establish a foundation of healthy eating habits, including a natural diet with fresh fruits, vegetables, healthy grains, meats, and good fats, use visualization as a tool to emotionally engage with your future self. Imagine yourself in your new body, wearing the clothes you love, feeling confident, and living the life you desire, also don't forget to include relationships, visualize who you would date or how you want your current relationship to be. Even better, you can even incorporate meditation to reinforce this new image of yourself.

Lesson Number 3: Avoid Negative Self-Talk

The words we speak about ourselves have a profound impact on our subconscious mind. Research by Dr. Masaru Emoto suggests that our cells react to negative thoughts, emotions, and even spoken words, especially yelling and screaming. Therefore, negative self-talk should be eliminated from your weight loss journey. Be mindful of the words you use and ensure they are supportive, encouraging, and positive. Treat yourself with kindness and compassion.

Another Observation

I've led many group fitness programs, which I called fitness boot camps. Back then, I was puzzled why the same two people of similar stature and likeness could start a weight loss program and one would get superb results while the other one didn't. Here's a great example.

"Sorry," She admitted sheepishly, "I'm late again, I know". I told her not to worry, to warm up quickly, and follow the others.

The next day she was late again, followed by frequent tardiness. She always had an excuse however, her car wouldn't start, there was lots of traffic, she felt sick, and her kids were acting up. I told her it was okay, as long as she showed up but I did wonder what was going on in her life. She always seemed hurried and in some kind of upheaval. Could it be that consciously she wanted to attend my group fitness classes but subconsciously she didn't? Bingo! And guess what, she didn't get great results with my program.

Why? Well, not only did she miss sessions or come late, she didn't do well with her meal plan either. When her time in my program was up, I talked with her about her experience and it was as if she didn't even expect to lose weight anyhow. She had kind of an embarrassed look on her face and said to me, "I never really lose a lot of weight but at least I'm getting stronger and healthier". I agreed with her to forsake an argument but really wanted to give her a lecture!

Looking back at this now, I could see that she was having a real internal conflict. She was trying to use willpower to get the job done but her subconscious feelings were contrary to the group fitness program she signed up for. What lessons can we learn from this example?

Lesson 4: Seek Congruence With Yourself

If there is a war between your willpower and your subconscious mind your willpower will lose every time. It's crucial to be in complete congruence with your weight loss goals. Kinesiology testing, such as the sway test, can help you receive feedback from your subconscious. I like the sway test because it's so simple. Use it to ask your subconscious if you really want to lose weight. Say something like. "I want to lose weight" and if you test positive, you are congruent with your conscious mind or willpower.

Lesson 5: Align Your Thoughts And Actions

If deep down, you don't truly want to take action towards your weight loss goals, you may unknowingly attract negative situations or circumstances that hinder your progress. At first, this may be hard to hear and it could seem like the one telling you this is insensitive but you do attract what you think about. If you find that every time you want to take action towards your health and weight loss goals you end up facing yet another unforeseen circumstance you could be sending out thought frequencies that are attracting what you really want. It's important to be clear and congruent in your intentions and actions. Monitor your thoughts and beliefs, and ensure they align with the steps you want to take. By cultivating positive and supportive thoughts, you can create an environment that promotes success.

Lesson 6: Foster Great Expectations

The final lesson we will extrapolate from our example is to have great expectations, as what you expect you will attract. Your expectations play a significant role in the outcomes you experience. When you believe and expect that you will achieve your weight loss goals, your belief will propel you toward the actions necessary to make those goals a reality. Set high expectations for yourself and have faith in your ability to achieve them. Believe in your capacity to reach your ideal weight and maintain a positive mindset throughout your journey. My client clearly did not expect to lose weight and she got what she expected.

So let me ask you, what do you really want? How much weight do you want to lose? Or let me put it to you this way. If I was to snap my fingers and give you the exact weight you wanted without doing any diet or exercise at all, what weight would you want to be at? What number would you take from me? Even if this number seems scary to you and unattainable write it down anyhow, because this is what you really want. We'll work on how to mentally, emotionally, and physically get closer to your ideal weight in the upcoming chapters. The pain you're trying to avoid is often where your breakthrough is.

Quick Recap and Action Steps

Let's do a quick recap before we move on to the next chapter. Recaps are good to reinforce and assimilate new information. If you want to reach your ideal weight, keep these six lessons in mind.

1. Focus on what you want, not what you don't want.
2. Embrace your power to change and visualize your desired outcomes.
3. Avoid negative self-talk and speak kindly to yourself.
4. Seek congruence between your conscious willpower and subconscious mind.
5. Align your thoughts and actions to avoid attracting negative circumstances.

6. Foster great expectations and believe in your ability to achieve your weight loss goals.

Action Step:

Get a journal and then write down the answer to this question. If I was to snap my fingers and give you the exact weight you wanted without doing any diet or exercise at all, what weight would you want to be at? Record this number in your journal and expect to get there!

Embrace self-love, practice visualization, and meditation, and monitor your thoughts to ensure they support your weight loss journey.

In the upcoming chapters, we'll delve further into techniques and strategies to support your mindset and help you overcome obstacles along the way. Remember, you have the power to transform your body and health.

How To Stop Making Excuses

Why You Have Difficulty Following A Diet or Exercise Plan

How come you didn't follow your meal plan this week? How come you didn't do your workout yesterday? How come you didn't follow your health protocol? Do you want to know the reply I usually get? "Chris, I don't know?" Generally, I shake my head and say something like, "You have to do better next time," although inside I'm kind of ticked you didn't do your part.

Have you ever wondered why it's so darn hard to stick to a diet or exercise plan? You know the drill: you start off motivated, but then you find yourself sneaking a cookie here and skipping a workout there. What gives? Why do we always sabotage ourselves? It's time to dig deep and unravel the mystery of our dieting woes.

Picture this: you're trying to follow a sensible, seven-day meal plan that supports your health, fitness, and weight loss goals. You know exactly what you need to do to shed those pounds, but for some reason, you just can't seem to stick to the darn plan. It's like there's a mischievous little voice in your head whispering, "Go ahead, have that extra slice of pizza. You deserve it!"

But why does this happen? Why do we fall off the wagon time and time again? Thinking about this behaviour used to really puzzle me until I found out the driving force was an Overweight Mindset and Emotional Blueprint. Granted, sometimes the non-compliant person had an excuse like:

- I had to pick up my kid
- Family comes first
- My husband was out of town
- I was sick
- I had a wicked headache
- I ran out of time
- I had to work late
- I was stuck in traffic
- I ran out of the ingredients
- My fridge was empty
- I can't cook
- I forgot

(Have you ever used any of these excuses as a reason for not following a diet or exercise plan? Smile right now if you have.) But here's the kicker: most of the time, we don't even have a valid excuse. We just don't do what we were supposed to do. The "Overweight Mindset" and an accompanying Emotional Blueprint are secretly running the show. It's like having a little devil on your shoulder, tempting you with excuses and derailing your progress. Sound familiar?

So, why does this happen? Well, here's the truth: it all boils down to mindset. Healthy-minded individuals always find a way to prioritize their health and well-being. They can juggle family, work, and their fitness goals like a boss. Meanwhile, those trapped in the Overweight Mindset believe they have to choose between their health and other responsibilities. But guess what? You don't have to choose! You can do both, my friend.

A Person With A Healthy Mindset Will Always Find a Way

If you often find yourself offering up excuses then this is an area that we'll need to work on changing. If you're the type to always come up with a laundry list of reasons why you can't achieve your goals, we've got some serious work to do. Healthy-minded individuals face obstacles too, but they don't let that stop them from taking action and getting the body they desire. On the other hand, those with an Overweight Mindset are masters of excuse-making, enabling them to stay stuck in their extra pounds.

Healthy Mindset people always find a way! They're like super-heroes who manage to juggle family, health, spouses, education, careers—you name it—and still, make time for their well-being. Meanwhile, the Overweight Mindset crew believes they have to choose one or the other. Seriously, folks, it's time to make up your mind and stop with the excuses. You can have your cake and eat it too—figuratively, of course—so let's get to work and make it happen! Make up your mind right now that from now on you will stop making excuses and do both! This simple action will help you to change your mindset for the better.

Are You Playing the Victim?

Have you accidentally slipped into a victim mentality? You know, the one where you blame your crazy schedule, your unsupportive partner, or life in general for your weight loss struggles. It's time to break free from that victim mindset and take charge of your own destiny. Trust me, tough love is coming your way.

Some weight loss seekers are really good at justifying their behaviour. They often tell me they're the victim of a hectic schedule, the victim of an unsupportive boyfriend or spouse, and the victim of family and work pressures. A victim of life! I know, you don't really mean to act this way but you do it anyhow because of unresolved emotions and your self-image. In my research, I have found that victims often leave clues. They have unsupportive behaviours surrounding weight loss which quite often shows up in these three ways:

- Blame
- Justify
- Complain

Maybe you're nodding your head right now, realizing that this hits a little too close to home. Perhaps you're that person reading this, struggling to take the necessary action to shed those stubborn forty pounds hanging around your arms, waist, butt, and thighs.

I hope you're still with me and I haven't offended you so far but someone needs to show you some tough love. You have to come to terms with where you are right now in your life. Remember, you cannot change what you won't or don't acknowledge.

The victim mentality is nothing more than the self-image trying to protect itself and remain the same. It doesn't want to change and usually defends itself in the forms of Blame, Justifying, and Complaining. It's not really your fault it's just where you happen to be at present. We'll talk more about the self-image in the next chapter but for now, let's take a closer look at the Victim Mentality and the games this mindset will play.

The Blame Game

Self-image defense mechanism number one is the Blame Game. The person stuck in this mentality will blame everyone and everything to try and remain the same. This person is often defensive and argumentative. It's always somebody else's fault why they are overweight. They will never accept responsibility for their actions. It's like they have a black belt in shifting blame!

Their spouse, kids, parents, previous weight loss programs, personal trainers, nutritionists, and even the high prices of healthy food become their scapegoats. They act as if the entire universe is conspiring against them! This person won't readily admit that there is something they need to change because they really don't want to change deep down. It's too much work! They know they need to lose weight for their health and a better quality of life, but staying put is just so darn comfortable.

This constant tug of war between "I want to lose weight" and the blame game will continue until they acknowledge this behaviour and heal emotionally. Once, however, this behaviour is recognized it can be corrected and the healing process can begin. It's time to step up, accept responsibility, and put that blame game on the bench!

The Justify Game

Self-image defense mechanism number two is the Justify Game. The person stuck in this mentality never likes to set meaningful weight loss goals. They think that losing ½ pound a month is okay and will justify why losing 1-2 pounds a week is not for them. This person sets goals so low that they can't fail and quite often they never really end up losing much weight at all.

This person likes to advocate that people should accept you for the size that you are even though deep down they desire to lose weight. This person is a master at offering up reasons why being overweight is okay and will rationalize why it's okay to maintain their overweight self-image. They pretend as if losing weight is not important to them and they don't really care about it. However, in most cases, anyone who says that losing weight is not important is usually overweight. In reality, this person is afraid of failure and finds it safer to remain the same than to embark on a serious weight loss journey.

Don't be fooled by all of these justifications. This person really wants to be at their ideal weight! Once they recognize this behavior, it can be corrected and the healing process can begin. They can then start setting meaningful goals and embark on a serious weight loss journey. It's time to raise the bar and show that they're capable of achieving more than they ever thought possible!

The Complain Game

Self-image defense mechanism number three is the Complain Game. Brace yourself, because this person is a certified crap magnet. There's always something wrong with them that prevents them from losing weight. And if nothing is wrong, they somehow manage to attract unfortunate circumstances that derail their progress.

Here's a secret: what you focus on expands. So, if you keep complaining and fixating on not losing weight or finding flaws within yourself, guess what? You'll keep attracting situations and thoughts that perpetuate the problem. This person is a champion complainer, always finding something to grumble about and engaging in negative self-talk.

But don't despair! Once this behaviour is recognized it can be corrected and the healing process can begin. They can shift their focus, flip the script, and start attracting positive circumstances that support their weight loss journey. It's time to break free from the complain trap and embrace a more empowering mindset.

Quick Recap and Action Steps

1. A person with a Healthy Mindset will find a way to do both.
2. A victim mentality has unsupportive behaviours surrounding weight loss which quite often shows up in these three ways: blame, justify, and complain.

3. Self-image defense mechanism number one is the Blame Game. The person stuck in this mentality will blame everyone and everything to try and remain the same.
4. Self-image defense mechanism number two is the Justify Game. The person stuck in this mentality never likes to set meaningful weight loss goals.
5. Self-image defense mechanism number three is the Complain Game. This person is generally a big crap magnet. There is always something wrong with them that is preventing them from losing weight and if something is not wrong with them they seem to attract some unfortunate circumstance that gets in the way of their weight loss results.

Action Step

In your journal come up with creative ways for you to do both the things that will support your weight loss goals as well as tackle any obstacles that are standing in your way. I would also like you to write in your journal what comes to mind when you think about the three victim mentalities. Is it possible that you've slipped into one? If so, which one?

Creating The New And Improved You

The Big Deal About Your Self-image

"I'm not a plastic surgeon", I replied. My new client wanted me to lift her breast, and her butt, she actually wanted me to make her butt bigger, (chuckle), her arms smaller, so they wouldn't giggle, and told me to make sure her thighs were no longer touching. I laughed at all of her outrageous demands! I assured her that I'll do my best but told her that I can only work within the confines of her genetic potential. I also informed her that her body works as a whole entire unit and is not selective as to where the weight will come off first. If I had known back then, what I know now, I would have also included some advice about her self-image as this is crucial information when creating the new you. At any rate, I'm happy to share this info with you today.

Your Self-image

Your mind is truly magnificent. From the moment you were born, it has been collecting data that shape who you are today. We call this your self-image. My simple definition of self-image is how you see yourself or how you perceive others see you.

Wikipedia has a very fascinating definition which I believe is right on the money. It states:

A person's self-image is the mental picture, generally of a kind that is quite resistant to change, that depicts not only details that are potentially available to an objective investigation by others (height, weight, hair colour, gender, I.Q. score, etc.), but also items that have been learned by that person about himself or herself, either from personal experiences or by internalizing the judgments of others. A simple definition of a person's self-image is their answer to the question "What do you believe people think about you?".

It further goes on to say that Self Image may consist of three types. We must gain further understanding of these three types if we want to improve or change our self-image. Wikipedia states that the three types are:

1. Self-image resulting from how the individual sees himself or herself.
2. Self-image resulting from how others see the individual.
3. Self-image resulting from how the individual perceives others see him or her.

These three types may or may not be an accurate representation of the person. All, some or none of them may be true.

I have underlined what I believed to be important in the last sentence, "may or may not be, some or none of them may be true". What I'm implying by the underlined fragments is that your self-image for our purposes is not true. A "Fat Self-image" is not supportive of weight loss and must be changed in order to have permanent weight loss results, in other words, to lose weight and keep it off.

Now, why is this relevant to your emotions and your Emotional Blueprint? Great question! Your self-image is heavily influenced or programmed by your emotions. It's like programming your mind with a specific set of instructions.

How You Were Programmed

Programming is what feeds or shapes your self-image. Just like you program a computer with data in order for it to do certain things. You were programmed from infancy to do certain things. You are basically programmed in three ways:

- **What you were taught** – this includes: hand me down beliefs from your parents, what you learned through media sources like TV shows, and magazines, what you learned at school, social and cultural beliefs, and the beliefs of your friends and acquaintances, small thinking from them that you hold up as truth.
- **The experiences you've had** – this includes: what you've witnessed and observed as a child, your experiences as a child into adulthood, especially the ones that have gone wrong. Not to mention, your experiences in relationships whether it's your boss, co-worker, friend, loved one, spouse, or boyfriend.
- **Behaviours that were modeled for you** – this includes role models or authority figures, anyone that we give power or major importance to in our lives. We tend to emulate their

behaviours, especially during childhood.

Interestingly, most of the beliefs and ideas we form as children solidify by the age of seven. So, if you were taught or experienced things that don't support weight loss—like constantly consuming processed foods or beverages your self-image got programmed accordingly. If you had really bad experiences like being severely punished by your father after misbehaving and then your mother in return giving you "comfort food" (usually processed food/junk food) to pacify you after your punishment then this bad experience programmed your self-image.

If you saw Mom and Dad sitting on the couch night after night eating potato chips. Guess what? You'll want potato chips too! The point is, when a well-meaning Health Coach suggests something supportive for weight loss, your existing programming may resist it. Your self-image is working against the very action we would like you to take.

Self-image Does Not Want to Change

Your self-image does not want to change. When you find your mind offering up excuses to not exercise or eat healthy it's nothing but your self-image trying to protect itself. You have more programming files in your head that support an Overweight Mindset than a Healthy Mindset therefore it's more easier for your self-image to stay the same than to change.

But fear not! Your self-image can be changed. By reprogramming your mind with more Healthy Mindset Files than Overweight Mindset Files, you can transform your self-image and overcome those mental barriers. But before we delve into that, let's take a closer look at your mind.

Stinking Fat Thinking

Now, you've probably heard the saying, "You are what you think about." Well, it's true! People with an Overweight Mindset tend to have unsupportive thoughts about their weight loss goals. They constantly say things like, "I'm so fat," "I have too many rolls," or "I'll never fit into that because I'm too fat." These thoughts originate in our conscious mind. When we attach emotions to them, they seep into our subconscious mind and become part of our programming—thus shaping our self-image.

Think about it. If you have a self-image of an overweight person, that's how you'll manifest in the real world. It becomes challenging to maintain a slim figure when your subconscious mind firmly holds onto the self-image of an overweight individual. How can you expect to become healthy and achieve your ideal weight when your deep-rooted programming revolves around being overweight? To fix this "stinking fat thinking," you need to consistently introduce thoughts of a healthy person into your mind and reprogram your self-image.

Your Mind Thinks In Pictures

Here's an interesting tidbit: your mind thinks in pictures. When you think of something, you visualize an image rather than words. For instance, think about the refrigerator you have at home right now. You won't see the word "fridge" in your mind;

instead, you'll see a detailed image of your own refrigerator. Fascinating, isn't it? This tendency to think in pictures can work to our advantage. By utilizing visualization techniques, we can reprogram our minds to adopt a Healthy Person's Mindset.

Your Roots

Now, let's talk about your roots. As my coach once told me, the weight loss industry often overlooks the importance of mindset work. Actually, his exact words were. "This Weight Loss industry is all bullshit! Nobody works on their mindset. They try so many different things and always gain the weight back because they don't work on their mind". I tend to agree with that statement. I wholeheartedly agree. While I believe I have the right approach to weight loss—such as natural nutrition, resistance training, and intense cardiovascular exercise for short durations—your roots must be changed to yield lasting results. Just like in nature, an apple tree's roots are programmed to produce apples, not oranges or pears. Similarly, if your roots are programmed to produce overweight "fruits," you won't magically produce a "thin" fruit. So, changing your roots is paramount if you want to produce the right fruit.

Quick Recap and Action Steps

1. Your self-image is crucial for transforming yourself.
2. It's how you see yourself or perceive others' opinions of you.
3. You were programmed through what you were taught, your experiences, and modeled behaviors.
4. Your programming and self-image influence your actions

and inactions.

5. Your self-image resists change because it's comfortable with the status quo.
6. Visualization techniques can help reprogram your mind to have a Healthy Person's Mindset.
7. The weight loss industry often neglects the power of mindset work, but changing your roots is crucial for lasting change.

Action Steps

Now, here's an action step for you: Find an old picture of yourself when you were much slimmer and had the body you desire now. The picture should be from around ten to twenty years ago, or as recent as possible. If you don't have such a picture, cut out the body you desire from a magazine and attach your head to it using tape or glue. Then, make it a habit to look at this picture in the morning as soon as you wake up and in the evening before you go to bed. Repeat this daily for at least 30 consecutive days, or until you notice a shift in your self-image toward that of a person with a Healthy Mindset.

Remember, rewiring your self-image takes time and consistent effort. Stay committed, visualize success, and watch yourself blossom into the healthy, vibrant person you want to be.

Emotional Eating And That Big Jerk

How Your Emotions Create Your Emotional Blueprint

"I'm gonna look so hot that every man is going to want me. That big jerk should have never left me, for that fat, ugly-looking, monster, he now calls his girlfriend! I want you to make me so hot that he regrets this! I want you to train me"! "Oooookay", I said, but what could I say otherwise, I could tell she was pretty heated and needed to blow off some steam. In this case, I knew enough to keep my opinions to myself. Just nod and agree, Chris, just nod and agree.

In retrospect, even though she was super motivated, this motivation was all wrong. It was coming from a place of, "I'll prove myself " and this type of motivation is always short-lived. Long story short, I did train her, she got a new boyfriend and quit her personal training. Go figure! Happy ending? Not really, she put the weight back on and if I was to guess, is probably in that same vicious cycle of seeking approval. You have to do it for yourself, ladies! You have to emotionally fall in love with yourself first, this is the best motivation!

Loving Yourself

You have to love yourself completely. Even if you're disgusted with the parts of you that are fat you mustn't reject it. Not only will you be unable to change this rejected part of yourself because you can't change what you don't acknowledge you will also create fragments of yourself. You will not be a "whole" person. When this happens you become emotionally unstable, unsure of how to act in different environments or situations. The part of you that is rejected will either be ignored, ridiculed or the butt of a joke. This will create shame or make you socially awkward in some situations. Because you hate parts of you you will also think that other people hate that same part of you as well. You will not feel comfortable in your own skin and you will find it hard to accept compliments from anyone. Not loving yourself completely will make it difficult for you to have relationships with others and yourself.

Have you ever gone to the mall not expecting to see anyone that you know, and then you see someone you know from work and you want to hide? This is an example of a fragmented person. Who they are at work is not the same as who they are at the mall. You should feel and act the same wherever you are and no matter who is present. This is what it means to be "whole". It's okay to be angry at your current predicament, the state that you've allowed your body to be in, no judgment on my end, but never internalize the anger inwards to the point where you hate parts of you or all of you. This is damaging to your soul and a setup for weight loss failure! Love is the most powerful emotion and you must be completely in love with yourself in order to lose unwanted weight and keep it off!

Your Emotions Are Glue

Emotions are really powerful and something I like to view as glue. Whatever you attach enough emotion to will cause it to stick to you, quickly get into your subconscious and attach itself to your self-image. I think emotions are largely responsible for programming many self-images. Think about this for a moment. (Remember my definition of self-image is how you see yourself.) When you are in a relationship with someone you are attaching emotion to another person using the emotion of love. In other words, you're gluing yourself to that person. This person gets into your subconscious, becomes a part of your programming, and now attaches themselves to your self-image. Have you ever heard anyone say, "I can't see myself without him". This person is clearly describing their self-image with the attachment to their relationship partner.

Why do you think relationship break-ups are so bad? It's because when you attach a lot of emotion to someone as in the emotion of love it bonds or glues you to that person and breakups become quite difficult because the self-image does not want to change. It will offer up reasons why you should remain in a relationship with that person. From the outside looking in we wonder why this person can't get over Johnny but to the person involved in the relationship Johnny is attached to their self-image and is presently their whole world.

Emotional Eating

A person with an Overweight Mindset does the same with food. Have you ever heard of the term emotional eating? I'm sure you have. This is when a person has a negative experience and then uses food for comfort. This experience with that particular food item or meal then causes you to release an emotion that you link or attach to that food item or meal. As a result of this emotional attachment the food item or meal gets into your subconscious mind, becomes a part of your programming, and attaches itself to your self-image.

Consequently, you visualize yourself with this unsupportive food item or meal often, which in return, makes it hard for you to stop eating it even though you know it's bad for you. You need to delete the emotional association of the programmed food item from your self-image to rid yourself of this emotional eating behaviour. This can be done by becoming emotionally involved with all-natural healthy foods that support your ideal weight and using EFT to clear emotions. A person with an Overweight Mindset will have a hard time staying away from junk food even though they know it will keep them overweight. Now you know why! In addition, the pain-pleasure principle is also another reason why people eat emotionally. Something I call your Emotional Blueprint.

Emotional Blueprint

Everyone has an Emotional Blueprint, your blueprint is your plan for moving you toward pleasure or away from pain. The definition of a blueprint is really a plan. If a plan is working for you that is an excellent plan; you'll want to use it over and over again. However, if your plan is not sufficient, not bringing about your desired results, you should scrap that plan or change it. In other words, your Emotional Blueprint is modifiable.

Everything that you've ever done has an attached feeling or

emotion to it. You've been collecting these emotions over time and they help you to decide what you would like to move towards and what you would like to move away from. All of the pleasant and happy experiences you'll want to move towards and all of the unpleasant and painful experiences you'll want to move away from. This is all factored into your plan and creates an Emotional Blueprint that you use to navigate through life. I should also point out that your Emotional Blueprint helps to shape your self-image therefore it's advantageous to recognize the blueprint you've created for yourself.

Are you getting this so far? Okay, it works like this, you have a thought, which leads to a feeling, you then consult your Emotional Blueprint for what you should do. If the feeling is good, you'll want to move towards it by taking action, on the contrary, if the feeling is bad you'll also want to move away from it by taking action. This entire process will eventuate into a result.

Where the problem lies for weight loss seekers, is when positive actions like eating supportive foods, that will cause you to lose your unwanted pounds are labeled as painful and you end up moving away from them. This is a problem because a healthy diet is needed for you to lose unwanted weight! When this happens regularly, you always end up avoiding the very thing you need to be successful. Even worse, it gets programmed into your self-image and you can't see yourself eating healthy foods. Another example could be a person who has wronged you, (painful) in response you use food to get over the offense. (pleasure)

Thoughts, Feelings, Actions, Results

When you find yourself in a bind and you're up against what seems like a gravitational pull towards that fast food joint you like, that sugary treat you like, that bowl of chocolate ice cream you like, or those bag of flavoured potato chips, just remember the acronym, T.F.A.R. This stands for your thoughts, that leads to your feelings, that leads to your actions, that lead to your results.

When your thoughts trigger emotions that are supportive, cause you to take healthy action, and create a positive Emotional Blueprint this is fine but when your thoughts trigger negative feelings or emotions that we do not want, we can correct this. We can do this by changing the original thought which has more to do with creating a new self-image to replace the old one. However, this may or may not be an easy task depending on the individual. Therefore it's sometimes easiest to start with the emotion or feeling that comes up generated by the thought. There are ways to clear negative emotions triggered by a thought so it no longer moves us to take undesirable action. One of the tools I like to use is called Emotional Freedom Technique or Meridian Psychotherapy.

Emotional Freedom Technique

The Emotional Freedom Techniques or EFT for short is a group of powerful processes that can help anyone be free from emotions that are causing problems in their lives. This highly focused energy psychology method allows me to release or decrease the emotional impact or charge of a feeling or emotion experienced by my client.

As a client brings their attention to negative emotions by way of thought I'm able to walk them through a process where they voice specific statements while tapping on a series of acupressure meridian points. With remarkable consistency, EFT reduces the level of stress in spite of the thought or remembrance of a situation being present. When the stress is reduced and the emotional charge is gone it is now easier to follow the thought with a positive action. In other words, EFT is a great tool you can use to change your Emotional Blueprint.

Stress and Your Emotions

One of the reasons why women can't lose weight is because they're too stressed out! A big source of that stress comes from negative situations, that trigger emotions, which in turn have an impact on our cortisol levels. As a Functional Diagnostic Nutrition Practitioner, I know this too well. Laboratory reports confirm that so many women are facing chronic stress and have elevated cortisol levels. Cortisol is our primary stress hormone produced by the adrenal glands. It is essential to help us adapt to stressful situations however when stress remains chronic and cortisol levels are constantly elevated this creates an environment where the following will happen:

- You gain weight around your midsection.
- Your digestive system is impaired and nutrient absorption is decreased.
- You have trouble falling asleep or staying asleep.
- Your immune system and nervous system are impacted.

- You have trouble building muscle.
- You have trouble losing weight.
- You have trouble with reproduction or infertility.

A body like this cannot lose weight! And that's not even all of the problems caused by stress and your emotions! However, there is good news! Regular EFT tapping sessions can reduce cortisol levels and prevent or reduce this stress response so your body is in the best environment for weight loss.

Several studies involving Dr. Dawson Church, PhD measured the levels of cortisol before and after tapping sessions. The study compared an hour-long session of talk therapy with an hour-long EFT session. The study found that anxiety and depression dropped twice as much with EFT and that cortisol declined by 24% in just a single hour. Can you see why I love using this tool with my clients and how beneficial it is? Using EFT to work on your Emotional Blueprint is the way to go! You can see my basic introduction to EFT by going here: www.coachwithchris.ca/book-resources

Quick Recap and Action Steps

1. You have to emotionally fall in love with yourself first, this is the best motivation!
2. Love is the most powerful emotion and you must be completely in love with yourself in order to lose weight and keep it off!
3. Emotions are glue and can be used to change your self-image.
4. Emotional eating is caused by the emotions you attach to

foods.

5. Your Emotional Blueprint is your plan for moving toward pleasure or away from pain. All of the pleasant and happy experiences you will want to move towards and all of the unpleasant and painful experiences you will want to move away from. This is all factored into your plan and creates an Emotional Blueprint that you use to navigate through life.

6. Remember the acronym, T.F.A.R. This stands for your thoughts that leads to your feelings that lead to your actions that lead to your results.

7. Regular EFT tapping sessions can reduce cortisol levels and prevent or reduce this stress response so your body is in the best environment for weight loss.

Action Step

Pick seven healthy foods that you can become emotionally involved with. Better yet, make them into a delicious meal. List all the reasons why you enjoy these foods and try eating these foods or making these meals regularly. Use your favourite song to create a pleasurable experience while eating your healthy foods.

Modifying Your Emotional Blueprint

How To Create A Winning Plan

She arrived at her appointment, "I ordered a pizza Chris", she said to me in a wimpy voice that sounded defeated. "What"! I exclaimed, "You were doing so well". She had lost twenty pounds with me, and now is back up five pounds over the weekend. In fact, she seemed to repeat this fiasco every weekend, sabotaging herself in some kind of way with food. I told her that she would have already reached her goal if she could only successfully get through her weekends. She then admitted to me that, she hated being alone, and ordering a pizza made her feel better. I didn't get it as much then but I totally get it now! Her Emotional Blueprint was hard at work.

Modifying Your Emotional Blueprint

In the example above we can clearly see that my former client had an Emotional Blueprint in place that said anytime you feel lonely, which was her pain, you must turn towards comfort food, which in her case was pizza, her pleasure. I'm sure this wasn't the only negative behaviour she suffered from but this was the one that routinely got in the way of her weight loss goals.

Your Unique Emotional Blueprint

As I stated in the previous chapter everyone has their own unique Emotional Blueprint comprised of emotional experiences. We can group these experiences into two categories:

- Pleasure – emotional experiences that will pull us toward a person, place, or thing that causes pleasure.
- Pain – emotional experiences that will push us away from a person place or thing that causes pain.

To discover what your personal Emotional Blueprint is I like to use the acronym, A.B.C. I'll explain below.

A: Stands for Awareness

You cannot change what you're not aware of. We need to make a list of all of the stressful situations and events that take place in our lives, especially those surrounding weight loss and body image.

B: Stands For Beliefs

You need to get rid of false beliefs. We need to make a list of false beliefs, especially those surrounding weight loss and body image.

C: Stands for getting clear

You need to clear problematic emotions and get clear on your future. We need to make a list of all of your negative emotions, especially those surrounding weight loss and body image.

Making Your List

You need to make a pain, pleasure list in each category to identify your Unique Emotional Blueprint. For example, you need to make a list of events, a list of beliefs, and a list of negative emotions surrounding weight loss and body image. This may require some help from a close friend or loved one you trust. Someone you can be yourself with. We also have group and private coaching where we walk you through all of these action steps and provide the emotional support you need for change. Contact me for a free session to learn how I can support you through this process by going here: www.coachwithchris.ca/book-resources

To help you start thinking in the right direction, I'll give you an example using an event. Let's say you used to date a guy named Tyrone, every Saturday morning you and Tyrone had this extremely delicious but very high-calorie breakfast, consisting of waffle cakes, topped with all of the fixings including, strawberry jam, syrup, and whipped cream, served up with eggs, fried potatoes, and sausage links. This is a memory that you hold very dear, you're reminded of him and feel very close to him every time that you consume this meal. Unfortunately, Tyrone is no longer with you, he passed away from an illness. This of course was very devastating for you but with time you've gotten over it, or so you think.

At work, your boss is a really big jerk, he doesn't pick on you all the time but when he does, he belittles you and makes you want to cry. You're angry inside, embarrassed, and stressed to the max. This is really painful for you and happens quite frequently, at least three times a week. You can't quit because you need the money. To cope, you come home after work and make that special breakfast you had with Tyrone to make you feel better.

Are you getting it so far? Your boss belittling you, is your painful event, and that high-calorie breakfast, that Tyrone special, is what provides you the pleasure. This is just one example, here are some things you might find on your events list.

Events List

- The boss is a jerk and he makes me feel stupid at staff meetings. I want to shoot him!
- Not enough help from hubby with the kids after school. I'm not superwoman, you know!
- My husband doesn't like my girlfriend Lisa, who tells me every day, makes me feel bad, and stresses me out.
- My mother-in-law is too critical of me, almost daily. She always stresses me out! She needs a muzzle!
- My daughter doesn't respect me and yells at me daily. Doesn't she know that I pay the bills? Ungrateful!

These are all the things that are stressing you out and should be on your events list. Feel free to add some detail, associating any feelings that come up for you. You'll also want to make a note of what you do to find pleasure as a result of your stressful event in a separate column. Some things people do when stressed out are: drink alcohol, eat comfort food, binge eat, smoke, have sex, take drugs, over-exercise, sleep, run away, and nothing. What might you do? What unsupportive behaviour is stopping you from reaching your ideal weight?

You can use the handout I've created from my Keep The Weight Off Coaching program to record your Emotional Blueprint by going to the web address below:

www.coachwithchris.ca/book-resources

Beliefs List

- I will never lose weight because everyone in my family is big-boned. It's in my genes!
- Losing weight takes too much time and is a big struggle for me.
- My momma said unattractive girls like me are overweight, only the pretty ones get to be skinny.
- I don't understand all this nutrition stuff.
- It's going to be too hard to diet, manage my meals, cook, and count calories. Who has time for that?
- I'm just not meant to be skinny!
- I will look too sick if I become slimmer.

Yes, yes, get it all out! Make a big list so we can change your Emotional Blueprint for the better. Don't hold anything back!

Emotions List

- I get so angry because I can't lose weight!
- I'm frustrated that I can't lose weight.
- I'm sad that everyone can lose weight except me.
- I feel hopeless.

- I feel losing weight is impossible for me.
- I feel bitter that I'm the only one in my family like this.
- I resent other people that are thin.

I should also highlight that judgments and associating pain in the body might come up for you as well, while you're working through your emotions list. Don't be alarmed if this happens, just write everything down in your journal. Judgments usually begin with the words "I am" and generally come from internalized emotions. Associating pain in the body and sickness can sometimes be caused by trapped or suppressed emotions, liken to a computer with too many files that starts to act up. For example, here are some judgments that you might have:

- I'm too stupid to lose weight.
- I am too dumb to lose weight.
- I am a loser.
- I'm not smart.
- I am ugly.
- I'm a retard!
- I'm a screw-up!
- I am fat and ugly.

It's no surprise that suppressed emotions can cause health problems. In Traditional Chinese Medicine, negative emotions are associated with illnesses in specific regions of the body. Check this out!

Health Problems Caused By Emotions

- Anger, jealousy, and envy can cause liver problems. This

can mean that the liver produces less bile, produces more cholesterol, and filters fewer toxins.

- Hate, cruelty, and impatience can cause heart problems. This can mean that you have heart palpitations, high blood pressure, and chest pain.
- Worry, anxiety, and mistrust can cause problems with your spleen, stomach, and pancreas. This can mean that you have impaired digestion, malabsorption, and an imbalance of gut bacteria.
- Depression and sadness can cause problems with your lungs and large intestine or colon. This can mean that you have breathing problems, less oxygen in the blood, problems with elimination, or constipation.
- Fear can cause kidney and bladder problems. This can mean that the body becomes acidic, you get frequent urinary tract infections, you have a lower sex drive, you have less vigor and your central nervous system is impaired.

Do you see how many things that can go wrong because of unresolved negative emotions? The body also does not let go of unwanted fat easily when you're unhealthy or not at your optimal levels of health. You have to get healthy first in order to lose weight Most people have this backward, they want to lose weight first then get healthy. Okay, so I wrote all that to say that your emotions are linked to your health. For example, here are some associated pains and illnesses that might arise when you work on your emotions list:

- Headache
- Stomach ache
- Diarrhea

- Lower back pain
- Chest pain
- Trouble breathing
- Feeling "choked up".
- Feeling dizzy

Congratulations! Give yourself a round of applause because you've just unlocked your very own Emotional Blueprint. This little plan of yours has been keeping you stuck in negative actions and, let's be honest, it's been a big contributor to your weight struggles. But fear not, my friend, because today is the day we kick that blueprint to the curb and embark on a journey toward your ideal weight!

I know, I know, it can be tough to dive into all this emotional stuff and make your list. But guess what? The hard work starts paying off now. It's time to claim your emotional freedom by making some kick-ass modifications to that blueprint of yours. We're going to strip away everything that's been holding you back and focus on unleashing the amazing person you truly want to be.

Are you ready for the transformation, my friend? Get ready to wave goodbye to the old you and say hello to the new, improved version! It's time to shine, to conquer, and to strut your stuff. Get those sleeves rolled up and let's dive in. The new you is waiting, and trust me, it's going to be a journey worth taking!

Modification Process

Now that you have your Emotional Blueprint on paper you're

simply going to rewrite your plan. You're going to change how you respond to events, you're going to change your beliefs and you're going to change your associating emotions, judgments, and physical pain, if any. In your journal, you are going to write down exactly how you want your life to go by basically jotting down the opposite of what you used to do previously. We're also going to use EFT or Emotional Freedom Techniques to neutralize negative emotions, reducing how they affect our stress response and cortisol levels. You can see my basic introduction to the Emotional Freedom Technique, EFT for short, by going here: www.coachwithchris.ca/book-resources

Here's where you will need some courage and effort as rewriting your Emotional Blueprint may seem scary to even fathom that such things could be possible for you! But guess what buttercup? Anything is possible for you! If you're wondering what this looks like here's an example of how you would rewrite your events list. Unfortunately, you're not in control as much, over the stressful events in your life, unless you remove yourself from the situation entirely, however, for obvious reasons, this is not always practical. You can, however, change how you respond to the event by associating positive pleasurable actions and neutralizing negative emotions with EFT.

Instead of Tyrone's special high-calorie breakfast as a negative pleasurable coping mechanism, you can replace this action with a positive one by taking a nice relaxing Epsom salt bath as a positive pleasurable action. This won't happen overnight but if we're intentional about it, we will be able to implement our new Emotional Blueprint and reap the benefits of feeling good inside and out.

You can use the handout I've created from my Keep The Weight Off Coaching program to record your Modified Emotional Blueprint by going to the web address below:

www.coachwithchris.ca/book-resources

Rewritten Events List

Here's what your rewritten events list should look like:

- My boss is still a jerk but that's just the way he is, probably because he doesn't like his life or has family trouble at home but he doesn't make me feel stupid anymore because I don't let him!
- I do what I can to help the kids settle in after school and no longer stress about what doesn't get done.
- I accept that my Husband doesn't like my girlfriend and continue to respect him but I also point out Lisa's positives so my Husband can see them too!
- My mother-in-law is still critical of me because she only wants the best for her son but I was able to set some healthy boundaries.
- My daughter thinks I don't understand her, so I try to look at things from her point of view and now we get along better.

By first neutralizing these stressful situations with EFT you're now able to look at your situations differently. As a result, you may no longer view these as stressful events, but even if you do, you have learned how to replace the negative pleasurable action with a positive one.

Rewritten Beliefs List

Here's what your rewritten beliefs list should look like:

- I can lose weight despite my family history and genes!
- Losing weight is effortless for me!
- I'm pretty and deserve to be healthy and slim!
- I have the ability to master my nutrition!
- I can easily manage my weight loss responsibilities!
- I have a right to be skinny!
- I will look amazing when I reach my weight loss goal!

Can you see how these beliefs are much more empowering? Do you get that these beliefs will pull you towards more positive actions? You can now use EFT to make these beliefs more believable for you as well as declarations. A declaration is a powerful act of speaking about what you would like to be as if it was happening right now. You can recite your new beliefs daily and use EFT to neutralize any negative emotions that come up for you while doing so. Both EFT and declarations will help you to execute your newly rewritten Emotional Blueprint.

You can use the handout I've created from my Keep The Weight Off Coaching program to recite some pre-written Healthy Mindset Declarations by going to the web address below:

www.coachwithchris.ca/book-resources

Rewritten Emotions List

Here's what your rewritten emotions list should look like:

- I feel happy that I'm losing weight!
- I feel joy that weight loss is possible!
- I'm happy that I can lose weight too!
- I feel on top of the world!
- I feel enthusiastic about my weight loss possibilities!
- I feel proud to join my family's body shape and size!
- I love other people that are thin!

You'll notice that most of this will happen by default as you start to look at things differently. You'll be able to replace skepticism, hopelessness, and despair with feelings of great expectation, love, and joy when you think about your body and weight! You'll also notice that some or all of your judgments have diminished and that all of your associating pains and illnesses are no more! You're on your path to true freedom in a body that you will love! You're on your path to your ideal weight without any fear that your weight will return! You're on your way to a new you!

Quick Recap and Action Steps

1. Your Emotional Blueprint is always hard at work.
2. Everyone has their own unique Emotional Blueprint comprised of painful emotional experiences and pleasurable emotional experiences.
3. To discover what your personal Emotional Blueprint is use the acronym, A.B.C. A stands for Awareness, B stands for Beliefs and C stands for Clearing and Clarity.

Action Steps

- You need to make a pain, and pleasure list using the categories: events, beliefs, emotions, and sometimes judgments and pain or illnesses, to identify your own Unique Emotional Blueprint. You can use the Emotional Blueprint Handout to do this.

- Use the Modification Process to rewrite your Emotional Blueprint.
- Use EFT and declarations to neutralize negative emotions and have a more positive outlook on life.
- You can find all of the handouts and see the EFT demo by going here: www.coachwithchris.ca/book-resources

Why You Shouldn't Surrender

Weight Loss Really Can Be Easy

After talking to many females I get the sense that they have just decided to surrender to unwanted body fat and forgo the pursuit of weight loss. I sometimes hear frustration, anger, resentment or even defeat in their voices. I began to wonder how did we get to this land of surrender? Why have so many decided to accept a body that they are not comfortable living in? The answer finally came to me.

How To Tie My Shoes

When I was just a little boy I desired to tie my shoes all by myself as grown-ups do. I would sit for hours trying time after time but the end result would be a bunch of knots in my laces that mother was not pleased to untangle. After countless attempts, I resented seeing my shoes and the laces and accepted that I don't know how to tie my shoes even though deep down the desire was still within. Then one day while watching Sesame Street (Kid's TV Show) I saw a simple shoe lace-tying technique that caught my attention. It looked so easy, I thought to myself, I could do that. After all, the example on the show was demonstrated by a little boy performing this technique right before my very eyes. I thought to myself, if he can do it so can I. I succeeded in tying my shoes that day and the rest was history.

Now you're probably saying, weight loss is more complicated than tying your shoe. My answer to you would be: it's not complicated but failed attempts can create complications. I get it, you've probably tried every diet and exercise program under the sun. You've explored more weight loss solutions than there are flavors of ice cream (and trust me, that's a lot!). But here's the deal—I know you're "diet tired," but let's shift gears and embrace the mindset of an overcomer. Let's give fat loss one last shot, shall we? I promise you, just like my final attempt at tying my shoes, you're going to succeed. Weight loss can be a walk in the park (pun intended) when your body is healthy and ready for it.

Now, if you've been following all the action steps in this book, it's time to crank up that optimism. You should be feeling more confident about your success this time around, especially if you've rewritten your Emotional Blueprint like a boss. But hold on a sec, we can't just leave you guessing when it comes to nutrition. It's like trying to solve a Rubik's Cube blindfolded—it's not gonna end well. So, let's have a little chat about weight loss and nutrition, shall we? After all, nutrition is the superhero responsible for 80% of the changes happening in your body. And hey, I wouldn't be doing you justice if I didn't practically walk you through it. So, grab a snack (a healthy one, of course), and let's dive into the world of nutrition with gusto!

Weight Loss Is Frustrating

Weight loss or better said, fat loss, can be really frustrating at times. There are so many diet programs, exercise programs, pills, potions, and lotions all promising you to have the body of your dreams. If this is your first attempt at fat loss you are probably still enthusiastic and hopeful of achieving your goals but if this is your 10th attempt or more I applaud you for sticking with me this far.

No Easy Way For Me To Tell You

Alright, let's revisit that little nugget of wisdom I dropped earlier. Remember when I said weight loss is a piece of cake for a healthy body? Well, here's the scoop: all those diets you've tried in the past, all those questionable food choices you've made, the junk, processed, and fake foods you've devoured—oh, and let's not forget about the toxins from alcohol, smoking, prescription drugs, and environmental pollution. Phew, that's quite a list! Unfortunately, all of these factors have turned your body into a not-so-healthy haven.

When your system is swimming in pollutants, your body's like, "Hold up, we've got some serious damage control to do!" And guess what? Fat loss becomes less of a priority. Instead, your body goes into superhero mode, wanting to protect those precious organs nestled inside you. So, what does it do? It cleverly uses your unwanted body fat as a hideout for those pesky pollutants and toxins. It's like your fat becomes their secret lair, keeping them out of harm's way.

I know it sounds like a comic book plot gone wrong, but hey, your body's just trying to keep you safe. It's got this "better safe than sorry" mentality going on. To make matters worse our bodies are not meant to digest what I call fake foods. These foods are processed foods and what we call "junk foods". Many of these foods have been manufactured by a team of scientists whose main focus is: the taste, addiction, and repeat business of these non-food items. What happens when you eat these fake foods over time is that it all goes in but not all of it comes out.

Simply put, you're eating difficult-to-digest food items that cling to your colon wall, wreaking havoc on your poor body. It's like a party gone wrong in your gut, causing pounds of waste to pile up, nutrients to go unabsorbed, and weight gain to run rampant. And let's not forget about the lovely side effect of constipation, making you feel like you're playing a never-ending game of hide-and-seek with the bathroom. Fun times, huh?

But that's not all, my friend. The consequences go beyond just a little tummy trouble. Your immune system takes a hit, your hormones start acting like rebellious teenagers, and you create the perfect breeding ground for sickness and disease. It's a messy situation, to say the least.

So, here's the deal. When your body is dealing with all this chaos, weight loss becomes a real challenge. Your body is like, "Hold up, I'm busy trying to keep you healthy here! Who cares about looking good?" And if I could channel your body's voice, it would probably say something like, "Excuse me? You've put me through all this junk for years, and now you want weight loss? Seriously?"

But fear not, my friend. We're here to clean up the mess, get your body back on track, and show it some much-deserved love. So, let's kick those fake foods to the curb and embark on a journey toward health and weight loss. Your body might just give you a high-five (if it had hands) for finally stepping up and taking charge!

Nutrition To The Rescue

Nutrition is 80% responsible for making physical changes in your body. Yep, what you eat holds more power than you might realize when it comes to shedding that fat and improving your overall health. Now, I'm sure you've heard this before, but it's time to take that common sense knowledge and turn it into common practice. It's time to walk the talk, my friend!

But here's the tricky part: the world is filled with a ton of misinformation, all thanks to those sneaky drug and food companies chasing after that almighty dollar. They'll do anything to sell their products, even if it means feeding you a bunch of lies. Canola oil, for instance, was once marketed as a healthy choice but turns out it's nothing more than a sly imposter. It's been oxidized, denatured, and definitely not something you should be consuming. And don't get me started on vegetable oil and all those other commercial oils lining the supermarket shelves. It's like a minefield of unhealthy choices out there!

Lies And Myths

As consumers of food, we've been told lie after lie after lie! This is why we're sick, diseased, and literally killing ourselves slowly with food. We're eating sick animals, sick plants, and other science experiments that are not real food.

We've been led to believe:

- Limit our fat intake
- Saturated fat and cholesterol are bad
- Meat from the grocery store gets an A+
- Whole grains are the best source of fiber
- That science is better than nature
- That cardiovascular exercise is the way to go for weight loss
- Supplements are bad for you.
- We need prescription drugs to stay alive.

This is only a small list, you can see what the wrong information has done over the years. It's made it difficult for you to lose weight, by no fault of your own, you have been doing things incorrectly time and again. Creating a compound effect of unhealthy habits that have held you prisoner in a body you are not comfortable in.

You may have even created a new identity around this heavier you. Dismissing a slimmer version of yourself as unattainable! And hey, I get it. It's easy to justify carrying around that unwanted body with excuses like "I'm too old" or a laundry list of other reasons you tell yourself. You don't have to settle for a life that doesn't make you feel good in your own skin. I'm here to show you the path to health and weight loss! I'll show you two methods of fat loss to get you into a body you're happy with. One method will be fast and the other not so fast but they're both great!

God Got It Right!

Not sure what your religious beliefs are but there is a chapter in the Bible that has this great list of foods that we should and shouldn't eat. The more research I do, it becomes clear why God chose the foods on this list. It is to basically keep us healthy and disease free! Regardless of your views on religion, you'll find there is an emerging number of health professionals, including doctors and scientists, that are coming forward with the same information I'm about to share.

Making Natural Food Choices

Time to start you off on the right path! I would like you to keep the following information in mind when making food choices. The food you eat should have no interference from man (i.e. processing). The food you eat should not be machine-made, as is the case with Genetically Modified Organisms (GMOs). The animals you eat should be grown, as they were intended to grow, and eat what they were intended to eat. This means that chickens should be free to roam and eat things like worms, insects, fresh grass, and corn and cows should eat fresh grass and other green vegetation, as they choose. Plants should be grown in healthy soil with good natural fertilizer, and free of all pesticides, herbicides, and fungicides.

Healthy, natural eating is pretty much common sense but as I said before my desire for you is that you make common sense, a common practice. Your home should have roughly 80% of foods that are not found in packages. For example, fruits, vegetables, and meats are generally not found in packages. (We don't consider meat as packaged foods) The other 20% will be things like bread, rice, dairy, spices, and condiments.

Common Food Mistakes

You have probably been led to believe that your diet should be low in fat, you shouldn't have butter, red meat, and eggs because they're bad for you and high in cholesterol. However, experts agree that ingesting these foods from healthy sources is extremely beneficial for your health. New research has proven that a diet high in cholesterol and healthy fats are not the cause of heart disease and related illnesses. The problem lies in the past consumption of sick animals, processed grains, and artificially manufactured foods like margarine.

Good Fats

If you have been led to believe that fat is bad, you have been lied to. Fats are extremely important for cellular function and hormone production. In addition, good fats assist in repairing cells, keeping arteries clean and triglycerides down. In many instances, a diet too low in fat is one of the contributors to an absent menstrual cycle or Amenorrhea, PMS, heavy cramping, and bleeding. Problems many women face today!

Good fats also help to metabolize the bad fats, they're good for your brain and will help your cells to fight inflammation. You want good fat on your side if you intend to be healthy and lose weight. The fats you should not consume are: pasteurized, homogenized commercial dairy products, cooking/salad oils like canola oil, vegetable oil, corn oil or roasted if nuts (the roasting denatures the fat in the nuts making it less healthy). We'll cover all the bad foods you shouldn't eat on the following pages.

Natural Proteins

Protein is responsible for multiple cellular functions, repair, and growth. Protein is extremely important, and generally speaking, most women should add (a little more) protein to their diets. As long as it's all-natural, free from hormones and antibiotics. In particular, the proteins we ingest from animals are extremely healthy, and beneficial and play a key important role in fat loss and muscle building. Be sure to have the protein in its natural form, meaning no need to take the skin off, and organic of course.

Natural Carbohydrates

I like to look at carbohydrates in two forms, fibrous carbohy-drates, and starchy carbohydrates. Fibrous carbs, for short, can be defined as your fruits and veggies, and starchy carbs, can be defined as your grains and root vegetables. Fruits and vegetables contain all your important healing nutrients and antioxidants. This should be the bulk of your diet. Starchy carbs, even though you will eat them less are not the devil but are needed for daily energy especially if you're very active. Also, when starchy carbs are adequate in your diet it will free up the job of protein allowing your body to use it for repair and cell maintenance.

That being said, grains are not as good for us to consume as they were back when our ancestors were alive. This is also why we are seeing an increase in gluten intolerance and related issues. Whenever we find an intolerance to something with our food, it is usually the result of interference from processing and added chemicals. Such is the case with milk and lactose intolerance. Therefore, it is best to stick with the root vegetables and limit the grains. So when you visit the grocery store, just remember we don't farm bread and pasta.

Quick Recap and Action Steps

1. If you give fat loss one last chance you will succeed just like I did at my final attempt to tie my shoes.
2. Weight loss is easier in a healthy body that has fewer toxins and pollutants.
3. Nutrition has 80% to do with the body making physical changes. What you eat has a bigger effect than you may think on your fat loss and health.
4. Fats are extremely important!
5. God got it right, eating natural foods is the way to go!

Action Step

For the next seven days try eating only natural foods as described in this chapter! No fake foods are allowed!

How To Eat Natural Foods

Using My Simple Eating System

Remember when I said there is a slow way and a fast way to get your body back into alignment and ready to release fat? This is the slow way, when I say slow I'm referring to a thirty to ninety-day commitment to see results in your waistline and health. This is all relative to the life you have lived up to this point. If you were really reckless with your body and consumed colossal amounts of junk and processed foods, boozed it up on the regular, and paid no attention to toxins then you're probably in it for the long haul. In contrast, if you were somewhat health conscious then thirty days should suffice to turn things around. At any rate, we're looking for 1-2 lbs of weekly fat loss in a thirty-day period. This would mean you can lose anywhere from 4-12 lbs using this healthy eating method I'm about to share with you. I call it My Simple Eating System. I called it that because I think if we're ever to eat properly again and stop dieting we have to go back to the basics and simply focus on eating real food.

Simple Eating System

This suggested 30-Day Nutrition Plan is for people who need a diet plan for eating naturally, and consistently. Following my nutritional advice will allow you to lose fat, achieve that flat stomach and improve your health. This suggested nutrition plan is not intended for the treatment or prevention of disease, not as a substitute for medical treatment, nor as an alternative to medical advice. Consult a physician or health care professional before you begin any new nutrition, exercise, or dietary supplement program. Use of any guidelines or recommendations herein is at the sole choice and risk of the user.

What You Should Eliminate

While following this simple eating system you should remove the following from your diet to get the best and fastest results:

- Sugar (sodas, pop, added sugar, sweeteners)
- Alcohol (all alcoholic beverages)
- Coffee (no coffee, drink tea instead)

How it Works

There are four food groups that make up the Simple Eating System. The four food groups are:

- Healthy Protein
- Starchy Carbohydrates
- Fibrous Carbohydrates
- Good Fats

These Foods Should Be Real

I can't stress enough how important it is to eat food as God or nature intended. The food you select from these four groups should be real or natural. The food you eat should have no interference from man (i.e. processing). The food you eat should not be machine-made, as is the case with Genetically Modified Organisms (GMOs). The animals you eat should be grown, as they were intended to grow, and eat what they were intended to eat. This means that chickens should be free to roam and eat things like worms, insects, fresh grass, and corn and cows should eat fresh grass and other green vegetation, as they choose. Plants should be grown in healthy soil with good natural fertilizer, and free of all pesticides, herbicides, and fungicides. Too many of us today are eating sick animals and sick plants and then we wonder why we are sick. "You are what you eat" would be a good saying to remember when selecting your food items.

Your Directions

Eat three large meals every day. Your meals should be spaced out every 4-5 hours or when hungry. Your three large meals will consist of a healthy protein, a starchy carb, a fibrous carb, and a good fat. 3 meals are best because they will trigger less insulin, increase HGH (human growth hormone) and help you to burn more fat. In other words, no snacking! If you want to burn fat faster you must trigger insulin less frequently and every time you snack you trigger insulin making it more difficult for fat release! You must also cut out caffeine, alcohol, and sugar. The only sweeteners allowed would be Stevia, Luo Han, Yacon, and once in a while, a little organic honey.

Measuring Portions

We won't be counting calories rather we will be paying attention to our portion sizes by noticing the serving size of each food item we consume. Healthy Proteins will consist of 1- 2 servings per meal. Starchy Carbs will consist of 1 serving per meal. Good Fats will consist of 1- 2 servings per meal and Fibrous Carbs will consist of 2-3 servings of fruit per day and/or unlimited vegetables per meal. It is very important that you stick to your portion sizes to make sure you get adequate amounts of nutrients and avoid overeating. Resist the urge to count and track calories as it's not needed.

What Is A Serving Size

Serving sizes for natural/unpackaged proteins, vegetables, fruits and fat can be determined by placing the item in the palm of your hand. It should be no bigger than the size of your palm. All other food items contained in a package will have the serving size on the food label. Get into a habit of reading food labels and identifying serving sizes when you go grocery shopping. Learn how to be a quick serving size identifier. This simple skill will amaze your friends. They will marvel at how your plate always seems to have the right amount of food from each food group on it. It won't be long before they start to emulate you!

What About Water

Water is great and you should drink lots of it however you don't want to deplete your electrolytes which are necessary for fluid balance in the body, energy production, and almost every major biochemical reaction in the body. 1/3 of your body weight should be consumed in water. To calculate this use the following equation: body weight X 0.333 = water amount in ounces. For example, the calculation for a person weighing 150 pounds is 150 lbs X 0.333 = 49.95 which we could then round off to get 50 ounces of water. In addition to this, we need to add 8 ounces for every 20 minutes of vigorous exercise and 8 ounces for every bad habit like caffeine or alcohol.

Treat Meals

Last but not least is your treat meal; as everybody needs a treat meal once in a while! I believe in 80% perfection, having a 20% allowance if needed, to relax from self-imposed diet rules. So have a treat occasionally! Treat meals allow you not to feel deprived and have hormonal benefits like increasing leptin and more leptin means a controlled appetite and a speedy metabolism. Two things we need on our side to lose fat naturally! Great treats are foods like pizza or burgers avoid or extremely limit sugary treats such as Twizzlers or M&M's candies, or any other kind of sugary treat. The more natural the food item the better. Also, try to stay relatively close to your portion sizes according to the Simple Eating System.

What About Alcohol

You cannot have it both ways, if you want to lose fat and have a flat tummy you must avoid alcohol. However, if you choose to indulge occasionally here are the consequences. Inside of you, alcohol equals 7 calories per gram, nearly twice the amount of protein or carbohydrates and it's the second closest to fat in caloric content. In a class by itself, alcohol can be absorbed directly from the stomach into the bloodstream without any help from the digestive system. Once in the blood it has no place to go, there are no friendly storehouses to welcome it like other foods; consequently it must be used as an energy or heat source by the body.

Alcohol goes to work so fast producing energy that other foods we have eaten aren't given a chance to be used as an energy source. They aren't needed while alcohol has taken over the job of energy production. So, the food that isn't needed just transforms itself into fat in hopes that it will be appreciated at a later date. End result, alcohol causes you to gain weight!

Examples Of Each Category

Below are examples of each category for beginners following this system to eat naturally. This is not a complete list and does not contain every available food item but is a good starting point for most folk! You also might want to grab my free PDF handout that has a more extensive food list. I'll tell you where you can get that shortly.

Healthy Proteins

- Organic Chicken and Turkey
- Wild Caught Fish-Salmon, Sardines, Mackerel..etc
- Organic Eggs
- Grass-finished, free-range beef
- Hunted or ethically sourced meats
- Spirulina

- Chia seeds
- Hemp seeds
- Maca root
- Amaranth
- Quinoa

Starchy Carbs

- Pumpkin/Squash
- Sweet Potato/Yams
- Brown Rice/Wild/Basmati
- Organic Corn
- Teff
- Beans/Lentils
- Buckwheat
- Millet
- Gluten-Free Bread

Fibrous Carbs

- Asparagus
- Bell Peppers (Red, Yellow, Green)
- Brussels Sprouts
- Cabbage
- Cauliflower, Broccoli
- Egg Plant
- Romaine Lettuce
- Spinach

Fruits (2-3 servings per day)

- Berry family-Blackberries, Blueberries, Strawberries, Raspberries
- Melon family-honeydew, watermelon, cantaloupe
- Apples
- Banana

Good Fats

- Raw Nuts and Seeds
- Coconut Oil
- Authentic Olive Oil
- Ghee
- Almond Butter
- Butter
- Avocado
- Plain Organic Grass-Fed Cottage Cheese
- (Not pasteurized)
- Organic Grass-Fed Greek Yogurt
- (Not pasteurized)
- Organic Grass-Fed Kefir (Not pasteurized)

Sample Eating Day

The following is a sample day using the Simple Eating System. Model this day for success and don't hesitate to shoot me an email at chris@coachwithchris.ca if you have any questions!

Breakfast

- Protein (1-2 Servings): 2 boiled eggs.
- Fat (1-2 Serving): 1 pat of butter for sweet potato, 1/2 an

avocado.

- Fruit (2-3 Servings Daily): 1 Serving of blueberries.
- Starch (1 Serving): 1 small sweet potato.

Directions: Enjoy 2 boiled eggs with a side of mashed sweet potatoes and half an avocado. Finish off your breakfast with a serving of blueberries.

Lunch

- Protein (1-2 Servings): 2 seasoned and baked chicken drumsticks.
- Fat (1-2 Serving): 1 pat of butter to top veggies.
- Vegetables (Unlimited): Steamed broccoli and cauliflower.
- Starch (1 Serving): 1 serving of wild rice.

Directions: Bake your chicken leg quarters. Enjoy your baked chicken and steamed veggies with a side of wild rice covered in gravy from your baked chicken.

Dinner

- Protein (1-2 Servings): 2 Pieces of seasoned baked salmon
- Fat (1-2 Serving): 1/2 an Avocado, raw butter for broccoli
- Vegetables (Unlimited): Steamed broccoli, organic tomato sauce
- Starch (1 Serving): Spaghetti squash

Directions: Enjoy baked salmon with spaghetti squash and organic tomato sauce along with avocado, and steamed broccoli covered in butter.

Note: organic tomato sauce is not unlimited as with other vegetables, because its a sauce you should only have 1 serving.

You Can Do It!

Follow this eating plan for the next 30 days and you will get great results. You can lose up to 4-12 lbs of body fat on this eating plan. If everything is right with your body you should continue this fat loss pattern every 30 days until you achieve your optimal weight. You will still see results focusing only on your diet however the results may not be as mentioned above if you're not keen to add resistance training, moderate cardiovascular exercise, and of course paying attention to the mind-body connection as you have learned in this book. Doing so will give you the best results.

For a more thorough breakdown of the Simple Eating System, you can grab my free PDF handout by going to the website address:

www.coachwithchris.ca/book-resources

Quick Recap and Action Steps

1. The Simple Eating System is for people who need a diet plan for eating naturally and consistently.
2. There are four food groups that make up the Simple Eating System which are healthy protein, starchy carbs, fibrous carbs, and a good fat.
3. Eat 3 meals every day with no snacks in between to keep insulin levels low in order to maximize fat burning.
4. 1/3 of your body weight should be consumed in water.

5. You don't need to count calories rather watch your serv-
    ings.

Action Step

Follow this Simple Eating System for 30 days to start the process
of healthy eating and a better you!

10 Day Fresh Start Juice Fast

Use Juice Fasting To Get Your Body Back

There is a faster way to get your body back in alignment so it will more readily let go of fat for you. I call it a Fresh Start. We all need a fresh start at times. I remember when I was a teenager I hated going to class. I found it rather boring and would rather hang out in the cafeteria playing dominoes with the boys or basketball in the schoolyard. Don't get me wrong I thought education was important and did excel when I was present for class however I failed to see why I had to be in attendance all the time. At least, that was my rationale at the time. To my surprise, the teachers disagreed with my logic and made this known to the principal. I was called down to the office and was told that I needed a "fresh start" at another school. Looking back at the situation now it was good for me to be away from the boys who influenced me to skip class. Let's look at this now in terms of your body, think about all you have put it through. Would you like to reclaim the health of your youth? Would you like to reclaim your figure? Would you like to let go of all the bad stuff in your body that's making it difficult for you to lose weight and is destroying your health? Maybe it's time you had a "fresh start".

How it Works

The 10-Day Fresh Start is a great way to get your body back and lose unwanted body fat. In these 10 days, you will be committed to juicing and drinking fresh fruits and vegetables to reset, recharge and restore your body. This will increase your vitality, vigour, and health bringing your diet back in alignment for optimal wellness. Now 10 days really is a short time but for those who are new to this, it can be a very dramatic change. If you wish you can start off with only a 3-day Fresh Start, however, if you have done a lot of damage to yourself and want to embark on reversing any illness in your body like type 2 diabetes or fibromyalgia. (Ailments I believe can be helped or reversed with this method.) You will want to extend your journey to 30 or 60 days. This length of time will require supervision by a health professional and your doctor if you're on any medications.

The 10-Day Fresh Start is not intended for the treatment or prevention of disease, not as a substitute for medical treatment, nor as an alternative to medical advice. Consult a physician or health care professional before you begin any new nutrition, exercise, or dietary supplement program. Use of any guidelines or recommendations herein is at the sole choice and risk of the user.

Juice Fasting Benefits

The 10-Day Fresh Start will do many things for you, below I have listed some of the benefits of participating in this journey to better health.

Eliminate Sugar Cravings

Juicing is a great way to give your body a fresh start and eliminate sugar cravings by flooding your body with an abundance of vitamins, minerals, antioxidants, and phytonutrients. Such fresh, clean nutrient dense energy will reduce and eliminate the body's need for sweets. This will also lead to reduced inflammation and increased energy.

Repairing Cells

Cells can become damaged due to an acidic environment in the body caused by eating too many acid-producing foods. Damaged cells are not properly able to excrete the buildup of toxic and acidic waste. Which leaves you tired and looking older. Juicing restores alkaline balance and enables cells to return to their ideal state. This leaves you with beautiful clear skin and a strong immune system that can fight off disease.

Alkalizing The Body

Acid gets stored in fat cells. It is our body's way of protecting our vital organs from damaging the body. Juicing alkalizes the body rendering fat cells less important. This leads to you being able to lose unwanted body fat more easily and creates an environment in the body that diseased cells do not like.

Weight Loss

If you are trying to lose weight, juicing will get rid of the waste in your body. Your body tends to store waste in your intestines which often ends up leaving you feeling bloated and heavy. Juicing eliminates waste from your body, makes you feel lighter instantly, and improves your digestive system. That being said, juicing is not a laxative. It is a natural way to eliminate waste from your system that leads to weight loss.

Directions

Each day you will have your juices from the recipes below for breakfast lunch and dinner. If you wish you can have a portion of your juice at the time of your meal and save the other half for your next meal. Be sure to drink plenty of water as well throughout your day. Herbal teas are permitted as well with a little organic honey or stevia to sweeten. Fresh Start Juice Recipes are below.

Breakfast Carrot

- 4-6 medium carrots
- 2 small beets with leaves
- 1 cucumbers
- ½ medium lemon peeled.
- 1-inch piece of fresh ginger-root
- ½ green apple (optional)

Juice the carrots, beets, cucumber, lemon, and ginger. If you decide to use apples, remember that they will add extra fruit sugar (avoid them if diabetic or hypoglycemic). Cut the apple into pieces and feed it into the juicer tube after the ginger. Stir the juice, and pour into a glass. Serve at room temperature or chilled. (Makes 2 servings, servings will vary depending on the size of vegetables and your juicer.)

Spinach Power

- 2-4 cups organic spinach
- 2 handful parsley or cilantro
- 6-8 medium carrots
- 2 stalks of organic celery with leaves
- 1 medium beet

Bunch up the spinach and parsley, and push them through the feed tube with the carrots, celery, and beet. Stir the juice, and pour into a glass. Serve at room temperature or chilled. (Makes 2 servings, servings will vary depending on the size of vegetables and your juicer.)

Juiceable Salad

- 4 romaine lettuce leaves
- 2 handful parsley
- 8 carrots
- 6 organic celery stalks with leaves

Bunch up the lettuce leaves and parsley, and push through the feed tube with the carrots and celery. Stir the juice, and pour into a glass. Serve at room temperature or chilled, as desired. (Makes 2 servings, servings will vary depending on the size of vegetables and your juicer.)

Sample Fresh Start Day

Repeat this simple schedule for as many days as you desire. (Drink water throughout the day and herbal teas if you desire.)

- Pre-Breakfast - Upon waking, drink a large glass of hot filtered water with lemon and/or ginger.
- Breakfast - Breakfast Carrot recipe or juice of choice.
- Lunch - Spinach Power recipe or juice of choice.
- Dinner - Juiceable Salad recipe or juice of choice.
- Pre-Bedtime - Drink herbal tea with stevia if desired.

Follow this program for the next 10 days and you will get great results. You should lose 5-20 lbs of body fat or waste from your body on this program. If everything is right with your body you should continue this fat loss or waste release pattern until your body has reached its ideal weight.

Quick Recap and Action Steps

1. Juice Fasting is a great way to reset, recharge and restore your body.
2. Juicing is a great way to give your body a fresh start and eliminate sugar cravings by flooding your body with an abundance of vitamins, minerals, antioxidants, and phytonutrients.
3. If you are trying to lose weight, juicing will get rid of the waste in your body. Your body tends to store waste in your intestines which often ends up leaving you feeling bloated and heavy.

Action Step

Try doing a Fresh Start for at least 3 days!

Don't Make This Exercise Mistake

How To Exercise Metabolically

Sue wants to lose weight. She aggressively does cardiovascular exercises five to seven times a week. Sue does 1/2 hr on the treadmill, 1/2 hr on the recumbent bike, 45 min on the elliptical trainer, and then tops it all off with a 1 hr long aerobics class. She maintains this routine for a couple of weeks and notices some weight loss. Sue's eating habits are okay but only eats 1-2 meals a day. Sue thinks doing weights will make her look like a guy, so she avoids it at all costs. Sue continues with her routine but finds it hard to stay committed to her taxing exercise schedule. Sue preservers and is thrilled with her weight loss. She lost 20 pounds! Great, Sue now figures I don't have to frequent the gym so often and reduces her visits to 2-3 times a week. She continues this trend and further reduces her visits to once a week. She finds herself gradually regaining the weight and is appalled to discover she is now 40 pounds overweight. Sue is dumbfounded as to why her weight came back so quickly. Frustrated, she revisits her initial seven days a week routine hoping to repeat past success. Sue wonders why her body is non-responsive the second time around. Sue decides to add more cardiovascular exercises to hasten her results.

The Big Exercise Mistake

Sue is making a big mistake! She is not exercising metabolically and doing too much "cardio" She lost some weight initially but sacrificed precious muscle in the process. Sue lost valuable muscle because of excess cardiovascular training and made no attempt to include resistance training in her program. As a result, Sue's metabolism slowed rendering fat loss a daunting task. Sue's excess "cardio", poor eating habits, and lack of resistance training were her downfall, despite increased efforts.

Please understand, Sue's super active energy-expending odyssey was doomed to fail. Once Sue decreased her cardiovascular activities her weight returned because she didn't have the muscle mass or metabolism to maintain her slim physique. So many women make this mistake. "Cardio" only routines are no good for permanent weight loss. What Sue really needed was good natural nutrition, metabolic training, and a proper thought life.

When You Do Too Much Cardio

When you do too much "cardio" you run the risk of losing muscle. That's why an aerobic instructor who doesn't make time for resistance training will be an overweight aerobic instructor. When you are exercising aerobically your body can use two methods of energy, glucose/glycogen which is more immediate fuel, and fat which is stored fuel for a rainy day. When you perform aerobics in excess your body's energy demands require all your glucose/glycogen. Your body's next step will be determined by the intensity of your aerobic efforts. If you're entire aerobic workout is intense your body can only use glucose/glycogen to handle energy demands. If your workout is moderately intense your body can use fat stores to handle the body's energy demands. If you perform long bouts of intense aerobics you will use up all your glucose/glycogen. When this happens your body is forced to find other methods of energy catabolizing muscle tissue, using amino acids as fuel. (gluconeogenesis)

An easy way to tell if your workout is intense or moderate is to use this simple test. If you can't talk or carry on a conversation then your workout is intense. If you're able to talk without gasping for air then your workout is moderate. Use this test to prevent your body from over-taxing energy demands.

Metabolic Exercising

Exercising metabolically doesn't rely on long bouts of aerobic training to be effective for your fat loss and/or cardiovascular conditioning however you will probably experience the most impressive results for your muscular, skeletal, and cardiovascular system using this method.

Unless you are training for a marathon the days of long periods of cardiovascular training for fat loss are over. Research conducted at the University of Tampa found that doing steady state "cardio" at a consistent pace that's not near maximal effort helps out with weight loss but only initially. This means that it's better for weight loss to select an exercise program that will allow you to reach maximum cardiovascular efforts such as what I teach in my metabolic training.

Doing A Little More Than Walking

Ladies, let's talk about walking. Now, don't get me wrong, strolling around can be great for some fresh air and relaxation. But when it comes to weight loss, it's like trying to catch a cheetah with a snail. Slow and steady won't win this race!

Check this out: a study in the Journal of the American Medical Association followed over 34,000 women and found that it takes a whole hour of moderate exercise, like a leisurely walk at 3 mph, just to maintain your weight. That's a serious time commitment!

But here's where it gets interesting. McMaster University did some fancy studies and discovered that a mere 18 minutes of high-intensity interval training per week can give you the same health benefits as five hours of slow and steady exercise. Yes, you heard that right! In just a fraction of the time, you can kick your metabolism into high gear and get those fat-burning engines revving.

So, ladies, it's time to trade in those leisurely walks for some metabolic training that will make your body work harder and smarter. Let's leave the snail's pace behind and embrace the cheetah within us. Get ready to torch those calories, boost your fitness, and make every minute count. It's time to unleash your inner fitness beast!

Great For Women Over 40

Metabolic training is very important for the female over 40 crew as it helps to increase the production of the hormone HGH which has also been called the "fountain of youth hormone". This hormone is in your body naturally but starts to decline as you reach your 30s. Studies show that high-intensity exercises like sprinting champion distance running for building bone density and muscle in women. This is true because high-intensity training prompts the body to secrete HGH or human growth hormone. Not only is this hormone good for building muscle and reducing fat it also rejuvenates connective tissue and skin by way of collagen. Exercising metabolically turns back the hands of time.

Great For Weight Loss

Exercising metabolically is great for helping you to reach your ideal weight while strengthening the entire body. My simple definition is: An assembly of exercises systematically put together to stimulate the most amount of muscle simultaneously while offering the occasional cardiovascular burst. Metabolic training is about engaging large muscle groups and performing exercises that utilize a variety of muscles at once. Metabolic training is about doing functional exercises and full-body movements that encourage strength. Seldom will we have muscles resting with this type of training. Continuous stress on the most amount of muscle is what we are after during our workout.

The Best Training For Women

As a woman, you may be wondering if this type of training is too intense or strenuous for me. Metabolic training despite its intense nature is safe for all ages. This type of training also only requires short exposure to be effective. This means that 20-30 minutes exercise routines are sufficient to achieve a fitness or weight loss result. Being in your 40s and beyond is not a reason to avoid exercise rather it's a good reason to start. In an article written by Dr. Mercola a senior health specialist, you'll find a list of benefits for beginning an exercise program in your middle years. The article is titled "40 Isn't Too Old To Start Intensive Exercise". I will summarize his key points below.

- Exercise prevents memory loss and helps to prevent the effects of aging.
- Women can reduce their fall risk with strength training and agility-type activities.
- Moderate exercise can reduce the risk of developing metabolic syndrome for those aged 55-70.
- Starting an exercise program will reduce or prevent premature death liken to giving up smoking.
- Unlike your sedentary friends, you will be 6 times less likely to die of heart disease.

Metabolic training uses bodyweight exercises, full-body exercises, combination exercises, and a variety of exercise tools to get the job done. You may be used to some of the tools used in this type of training like kettlebells and dumbbells however because I specialize in the over-40 female crowd I have developed specific exercises and devices not normally used for training. I have developed some unique exercises to address female areas of concern while taking into consideration exercises to improve balance, core strength, bone density, healthy joints, and anything deemed important for your advancing years. The metabolic training that I specialize in addresses key areas of fitness that women over 40 should be able to perform.

What I'm noticing with most women over 40 is that the glutes or buttocks are severely underdeveloped which is a reason why the majority of females I meet cannot squat properly. The thighs are weak, particularly around the knee joint. This is due to improper exercise form or a lack thereof. The upper body is non-existence due to neglect and basic flexibility, coordination and motor skills are fading.

A big mistake made by women over 40 is thinking that they are too old to exercise. Ignorance towards metabolic training and fear prevent women from participating in other exercises besides cardio and yoga. I like yoga and believe it's beneficial but it should be in addition to and not in replace of metabolic training. Yoga has its own great benefits but you will forgo the myriad of health benefits mentioned earlier if you omit metabolic training from your wellness plan.

Moving Naturally

Metabolic training is about moving naturally and exercising the body as a whole unit. It's not about spot conditioning as you cannot spot condition fat. If the back of your arms requires toning and you only perform arm exercises, the flab will still remain. If your buttocks and thighs need reducing and all you ever do is use the leg extension machine at the gym, then I'm sorry but nothing will ever change for you. Your body works as a whole entire unit. If you want to shed fat and tone then you must work your body as a whole entire unit.

Your body stores fat in multiple fat stores. Your body only burns fat in designated fat-burning zones otherwise called your muscle. The good news is you can determine how many fat-burning zones you have. Developing muscle all over your body in addition to paying attention to target areas is fundamental to having the body you desire. Trying to rid fat from your stomach by only performing crunches will give your body only one fat-burning site. Not effective for weight loss or the area you are targeting.

The fat deposited around your stomach and vital organs is called visceral fat. Visceral fat is very unhealthy and is associated with heart disease, high blood pressure, stroke, diabetes, and breast cancer. Visceral fat is more common in men. Fat located under the skin is called subcutaneous fat. This is more common in women generally distributed in the hips and thighs. Although, subcutaneous fat carries less risk because as it is not surrounding vital organs, excess storage can potentially lead to cellulite. High-intensity exercises such as those I teach in my metabolic exercise programs will cause fat to be released into the bloodstream and burned at your multiple fat-burning sites (muscle). Insufficient muscle mass makes for poor metabolization of fat.

Swinging a kettlebell with proper technique is a great metabolic exercise. It involves multiple muscle groups at once and is one of the many tools I use to develop your metabolic training programs.

Quick Recap and Action Steps

1. "Cardio" only routines are no good for permanent weight loss.
2. When you do too much "cardio" you run the risk of losing muscle.
3. Unless you are training for a marathon the days of long periods of cardiovascular training for fat loss are over.
4. Studies at McMaster University suggest that 18 minutes of high-intensity interval training per week can deliver many of the health benefits of five hours of sustained moderate exercise.
5. Metabolic training is very important for women over 40 as it helps to increase the production of the hormone HGH.
6. HGH or human growth hormone is good for building muscle and reducing fat it also rejuvenates connective tissue and skin by way of collagen.
7. Exercising metabolically turns back the hands of time. My simple definition for Metabolic Training is: An assembly of exercises systematically put together to stimulate the most amount of muscle simultaneously while offering the occasional cardiovascular burst.
8. Being in your 40s and beyond is not a reason to avoid exercise rather it's a good reason to start.
9. Metabolic training uses bodyweight exercises, full-body exercises, combination exercises, and a variety of exercise tools to get the job done.
10. A big mistake made by women over 40 is thinking that they are too old to exercise.
11. Metabolic training is about moving naturally and exercising the body as a whole unit.
12. You cannot spot conditioned fat.

Action Step

Make sure your next workout is a metabolic one!

Living Your New Healthy Life

How To Live Your Best Life

Simply put, when I think back to all the thousands of clients I have helped over the years. The ones who lost weight the quickest with me had a Healthy Mindset backed by a supportive Emotional Blueprint. These people, if I were to run into them again, at the mall or grocery store, are probably still in shape to this very day.

Others who've lost weight with me in the past didn't start out with a Healthy Mindset, but I believe in time they developed this mindset accidentally. While others lost weight during our time together but have gained it all back because they only had a slight mindset shift.

Some People did not lose weight with me at all. They may have had some positive body responses here and there but the Overweight Mindset was never changed and their Emotional Blueprint was still directing them so their results were insignificant.

Is it all about your Emotional Blueprint, self-image, and Overweight Mindset? Yes and No! You can't help what you were taught during childhood and you can't help all of your experiences up until now but you do have a choice going forward to make some positive changes in your life to take actionable steps that will lead you in the direction you want to go.

You Can't Just Think Thin

You can't just think your way thin! That will never happen, you must have a diet that contains real food, as nature intended. Healthy proteins, healthy fats, healthy fruits, and vegetables, including healthy grains. You must eat when you're hungry and drink when you're thirsty. This will vary for everyone based on your dietary preferences, location, culture, and lifestyle. There is no one perfect diet for everyone or one diet that trumps the rest. The diet that is currently working for you, that encourages you to eat healthy, real foods, not processed foods or non-foods, that allows for 20% error is a diet that I would encourage. You can achieve your ideal weight on any diet that has these principles!

Exercise Philosophy

You must also move often, not out of fear or vanity but because you enjoy it. If you love the gym then go but if you don't, do something else that requires movement. Your body doesn't really care what you do as long as you do it! Dance, yoga, swim, bike, play games, sports, walk, run, you have ample opportunities to move often, so just do it. Develop good habits and routines based on the type of body you're after. Just know that for every goal or body type you seek there will be an accompanying amount of labour that is required to get there and also, maybe a change in diet but the choice is yours. You get to decide how you want to look and feel. Nobody can take this away from you!

Loving Your Life

Nevertheless, there are consequences, if you have neglected your body for a long time, by way of eating poorly, not moving regularly, and suppressing your emotions. You may have to work extra hard to undo the conundrum you've gotten yourself into. Which just means it may take you longer to reach your ideal weight. This has nothing to do with your blood tests being normal because the doctor could miss things. This has nothing to do with you getting older because your body still responds when you make it healthy and love it up. This has nothing to do with eating less and exercising more or else the millions of women doing this would've become slim by now. This only has to do with completely loving life, and doing positive things for your mind, body, and soul that will build health on a regular basis!

Loving Yourself

If you love yourself you will give your body all the things it needs to be healthy. You will nourish it with only the best foods, water, herbs, and spices. You will surround yourself with uplifting people and the things that sing to your soul, and spirit and make you feel joy. You will have healthy boundaries, you won't allow yourself or others to treat you badly or talk to you any way that they feel. You will move often because it tones up your muscles, gets your heart pumping, and makes you feel sexy. You will set goals without limitations and go after the body you want because that's how you want your body to look! This is the body that makes you feel good and how you want to present yourself to the world!

Freeing Yourself

Above all, what I want you to get from this book is freedom. I truly want you to be free from the negative mental prison and emotions that are keeping you in an uncomfortable body and a fragmented soul. I want you to be completely whole as a person and I don't want you to harbour toxic emotions and feelings that keep you overweight and unhealthy, rather I want you to express yourself fully. You see, at times, the unwanted weight you carry around on your body is merely a symptom of you not being able to become all that you want to be.

Somewhere along your journey in life, someone told you that you would be no good at your passion, you're not smart enough to become your desire, you don't have the body to wear that dress, you're not pretty enough to date me, you're not sexy enough to be my wife, you're not fit enough to do this exercise, you're not educated enough to earn this kind of money, you will never accomplish your dreams, yada, yada, yada and the list goes on and on.

You believed all of these lies that were fed to you and what probably sucks even more, is that the bearer of bad news was most likely coming from someone you loved, cared about, or respected in some way. Maybe the offending party was a spouse, boyfriend, parent, friend, teacher, or bully.

Suppressed Emotions

Indoctrinated with these lies, you wanted to become invisible, you wanted to shrink, and you ceased to express yourself. The accompanying behaviour, as a result, was that you withdrew from people and perhaps from life. You began to suppress your true self, your emotions, and your inner desires.

What you suppress long enough turns to depression and depression leads to sickness, disease, and weight gain. At this point, people usually turn to food for comfort, anti-depressants, or other recreational drugs like alcohol that do the same thing. When lack of expression is dealt with using food or drugs it's really upsetting because the end result is often increased depression, more weight gain, and a dampened self-image. A vicious cycle!

What you really must do is fix it. Fix your life! Avidly go after the body, health, and desires of your heart. Perhaps you're functioning at half of your potential and have settled for success in certain areas of your life but I want you to know that you can have it all. You are in control of everything you want to be, do, and have, no one else. Never let anyone stop you! Never let anyone cause you to shrink or suppress your dreams!

Express Yourself

Everything in nature is seeking greater expression and fuller expansion and you my friend are a part of nature. An acorn desires to become an oak tree and it does. Your desire to become whatever it is that you feel led to become should be just as simple as the acorn's manifestation; so why don't you just go out and do it!

I know what you're thinking, you probably don't even know where to begin. What you should do or how you should start to express yourself. Even worse, you might not even feel that you have permission to go after the body, health, and weight you really want. That's why I really want you to read through this book a second time and complete all of the exercises.

Work on clearing your negative emotions, improving your self-image and mindset, rewriting your Emotional Blueprint, and getting support. Surround yourself with people who want you to become your true authentic self. When you get rid of all of the unconscious junk that is standing in your way not only will you reach your ideal weight but you'll begin to come alive!

Coming Alive

It's time for you to become fully alive, to live the life that you desire without apologies, hesitations, or reservations. It's time for the real you to step forward, not the one you've been presenting to the world, that's all covered up. Are you ready to come forward? Are you ready to move away from unwanted weight? Are you ready to be free from emotions that are not serving you? All you have to do is make a decision, you can do, be and have anything you want! I love you and know you can do it! Go for it!

Quick Recap and Action Steps

1. True weight loss requires a Healthy Mindset backed by a supportive Emotional Blueprint.
2. If you keep gaining the weight back it could be because you only had a slight mindset shift.
3. It's not all about your Emotional Blueprint, self-image, and Overweight Mindset but you are responsible for your choices going forward.
4. You can't just think your way thin! That will never happen, you must have a diet that contains real food, as nature intended. Healthy proteins, healthy fats, healthy fruits, and vegetables, including healthy grains.
5. There is no one perfect diet for everyone or one diet that trumps the rest. The diet that is currently working for you, that encourages you to eat healthy real foods, not processed foods or nonfoods, that allows for 20% error is a diet that I would encourage.
6. You also must move often, not out of fear or vanity but because you enjoy it.
7. There are consequences, if you have neglected your body for a long time, by way of eating poorly, not moving regularly, or suppressing emotions. You may have to work extra hard to undo the conundrum you've gotten yourself into. Which just means it may take you longer to reach your ideal weight.
8. If you love yourself you will give your body all the things it needs to be healthy.
9. At times, the unwanted weight you carry around on your body is merely a symptom of you not being able to become all that you want to be.

10. What you suppress long enough turns to depression and depression leads to sickness, disease, and weight gain.
11. When you get rid of all of the unconscious junk that is standing in your way not only will you reach your ideal weight but you'll begin to come alive!

Action Step

It's time for you to feel fully alive, to live the life that you desire without apologies, hesitations or reservations. Write down all the ways you will start to express yourself. Write down three ways you can become more alive!

A Message From Your Body

Encouragement From Your Future Self

Hello, this is your body, you may find this quite weird but I urgently needed to speak with you. We know each other quite well and have been through a lot together. We have shared some good and bad times. I love you very much but there are moments when I question if you love me. Many times I have tried to get your attention but you are too busy to notice my signals. I have given you countless hints and have even tried to speak with you through others. My last resort was to write you this letter in hopes that the very act of reading will cause you to slow down and focus on what I have to say.

I'm writing you from the future. For your protection, I'm forbidden to inform you of the date and year. I know you have been trying to take care of me. I recognize your efforts. Likewise, I have been trying to take care of you. I have been working day and night to quarantine and eliminate illness from us but I keep being inundated with the wrong stuff. I can no longer do this on my own. I need your help. I'm left with no other option but to just come out and tell you what I need from you.

We have much left to do together. There are so many big things in store for your future. The problem I'm having with you is there is a great deal more you need to learn to take care of me. I need to move more often. I need to be nourished better with foods that are pure. I need to breathe clean air and have hydration from immaculate water. I need you to have more concern for me. In other words, I need you to step it up big time!

If not, you are going to run into some serious problems. Yes, you will encounter huge obstacles with me if you don't start making some changes. You must improve your motivation for health. You must be relentless in taking care of us. You must be consistent, you must be accountable. You must persevere.

You are going to be tremendously successful if you are relentless! Not only with your health but with everything you attempt to do. Remember what I am saying when you feel like giving up. Remember these words when you feel like quitting on us. Be inspired by this letter the next time you face a challenge you are not up to. Keep taking action! Press on! Keep moving forward because abundant health and greatness await you!

Be courageous and act in spite of fear. Find people and tools to support us. Keep taking small steps in the right direction. You have already done so much, I know. Let us now go to that next level of health. Let us be victorious. It's going to be incredible and I hope you can make it. I hope you can make us better. See you in a few years, my friend. I love you!

Sincerely,

The Future You

Chris's Motivational Quotes

Encouragement And Inspiration From Chris's Quotes

Below you will find a collection of my quotes for you to read through. Visit them when you're feeling a bit down or to reinforce positive thinking.

- Diet and exercise alone will not get rid of emotional weight.

- When you're healthy in mind and body weight loss is easy.

- You can't dwell on failure and produce a positive result.

- Trapped emotions can prevent weight loss.

- More of the wrong thing isn't better.

- You must have confidence to pursue the dream in your heart.

- If you make a change in your beliefs then your behaviour changes.

- Great achievers learn to replay the memories of their past successes, not failures.

- You are designed to be happy so be happy.

- By changing your mind you change everything.

- You cannot live beyond your belief system.

- Solve your problems and get results, ignore them and get none.

· You will always move towards your most dominant thought.

· Your body was designed to heal itself.

· Slow down, take time to rest, and love yourself.

· An investment in health will keep on giving returns.

· You keep doing the same thing over again and losing, change it up so you can win.

· If your body is not changing that doesn't mean you should exercise harder.

· Decisions make the difference between disappointments and destiny.

- Eek mutating cells are making you sick.

- Do not invest all of your energy in others.

- Do not endure what you can cure.

- True health is taking charge of your internal and external environments.

- Make your cells healthy and you will be too.

- Build your health from the inside out.

- You deserve to be the best version of yourself.

- Make yourself a priority.

- Great health requires preparation.

- Proper management of your health is better than prayer.

- If you manage your health well you will always have more.

- Don't push your body harder than you want to push your nutrition.

- A victim will always have poor health but the one who takes responsibility changes things.

- If you want to change your health you must change your thinking and sometimes your friends.

- No one can take you farther than you believe you should go.

- Our bodies are organic and not synthetic, we need things that are organic and not synthetic.

- You have the power to change your health today.

- Whatever you mismanage you lose, this also applies to your health.

- Growing old is optional.

- Every food from our creator is good for us but not every food is right for each individual.

- Exercise without proper nutrition is bad for you.

- Most women don't like to talk about their weight because they feel they have no power over their circumstances but the opposite is true.

- If you don't design your health somebody else will.

- If you want to die fast try helping everyone.

- Sometimes we do enough to relieve a guilty conscience but not enough to change.

- Nature's food gives you nourishment, naughty food gives you nothing.

- Our bodies break down not because we're old but because we're deficient in nutrients.

- Not eating vegetables will slow your weight loss.

- A life without vegetables is like a kitchen without a knife.

- To change you've got to stop listening to the same voices playing over and over again in your head.

- We not only pay for what we do in life but also for what we do not do.

- You can't be overweight and healthy at the same time.

- Knowledge breeds confidence but so does love.

- If you're feeling icky you're not operating in love.

- If you do not love yourself your health will suffer.

Praise From Clients

Past Results From Happy People I've Helped

I've loved that Chris and his team create an environment where anybody in any shape can feel comfortable and confident making this type of change. Since starting I've found myself to be more centered, balanced, and motivated in all aspects of my life. I've more energy for my kids, my work and have even secured a promotion within my organization. With this program I see results that make me actually want to look in the mirror for the first time in about seven years, I've lost over 30 lbs, more than 10 percent body fat and I just feel good about myself. I'm not the size I'd like to be just yet but I can already tell that by continuing to come and making this commitment to myself that I will get there much more quickly than had I elected to join a gym or try it on my own. Thanks, Chris, for my current success and for helping me to attain my goals.

-Sarah

Hi Chris, Thank you so much, for being such a wonderful human being. I have lost 12 pounds within 29 days I am super excited. I am now one size smaller..my body is definitely tighter and more defined. My tummy has definitely shrunk as well ..I have a way to go, this has become a lifestyle for me. I plan to be living healthy for the rest of my life. Yesterday I took a good look at my body, and really like what I saw, that feeling I got looking at myself, continued as I was walking outside, for the first time in a long time, I realized that I Angella Gill love my body. I mean it is not exactly the way I want, after all, I am a woman, lol, however, I do love my body, and it is going to get better every day as I work at it, work out and eat healthy. So thanks again.

-Angella

After an exceptionally challenging month, I am happy to end this month on a higher note. I am feeling better, I'm less tired and a visit to my naturopath yesterday confirmed it – my thyroid is normal, my adrenals are good, and I'm cleared to exercise again. I even dropped 4 pounds! Thanks, Chris for all the support!

-Tia

Thank you, Chris Walker! I did it!!! I feel great... I have changed my eating habits, my energy level has increased. I go to the grocery store and get the healthy food! My kids are eating better. I count my steps during the day. I have lost 12.5 lbs so far and I am determined to keep going thanks to you!

-Regan

I have been training for only 7 weeks now and have already lost 12 lbs, 6% body fat, and several inches...EVERYWHERE! More than anything I enjoy that I have energy again. Instead of sitting on the couch eating chips I now actively enjoy time with my family going for walks or bike rides. I still have a long way to go to meet my final goal but with Chris's help, I know I can't fail! Thank you Chris! Sincerely,

-Theresa

Thank you Chris for your help in making me lose weight because of you you made my heart healthy and you gave me a gift of happiness, joy of eating, and fitness for life I am forever grateful of you and your program Thanks

-Sophia

Chris, I want to thank you from the bottom of my heart. You have truly been an inspiration and learning experience. I have dreaded every Monday, Wednesday, and Friday at 8 am, haha. A love-hate relationship. You have been such a positive life-changing aspect in our life. A pleasure to work with. You are a good soul, Bless You.

-Lori

I worked with Chris who taught me the importance of a LIFESTYLE rather than what I have done before, "a calorie-counting diet" that simply didn't last. Chris worked with me and showed me what I needed to do, eat, etc... and help me shed 34 pounds! As a result, I feel better about myself, and my life, and find it easier to tackle the tough things in life. Thank you, Chris! Anyone thinking about getting in shape but is making excuses, (can't find time, can't, can't, can't) and want to take control over their life, give him a call!

-Jon

Thank you, Chris!!! You have helped me improve my overall health. Before going through this 30-day challenge: I ate too much, I ate the wrong types of foods, I had low energy, I felt tired throughout my day, I was not happy with my body. Things I have learned during this journey: The correct potion sizes for my meals, How to eat healthily, How to stop my cravings, and How to change my mindset. How this journey has changed my life: I have lost 20 lbs. My start weight was 218 lbs and I now weigh 198 lbs, I have energy from food, I no longer feel tired during the day, I am excited to continue on this journey of healthy living, I have stopped drinking coffee. I used to drink two to three cups a day (double, double), I have stopped eating comfort foods, I have a support chain to help me stay on track, I am 100% committed to staying focused on healthy choices and including exercise in my day. My menstruation cycle has improved (See Chris Walker's posting "Eliminate Estrogen Dominance). I used to have heavy bleeding, headaches, and cramping. By changing what I eat I now have a normal menstruation cycle. This has been a wonderful experience. My overall health has improved. I am looking forward to working with Chris over my journey to attain my BMI goal and overall health.

-Nancy

I started the 30-day challenge with Chris Walker at an all-time high weight for myself of 241 lbs. I had not taken very good care of myself physically or paid attention to my eating habits for years. I would usually consider a short walk as my exercise for the week. Fast food had quickly become my go-to meals. I didn't have much hope when I started the challenge that it would work for me as not many other diet/exercise plans had in the past. Following the meal plan and incorporating the exercises from Chris was a lot simpler that I had realized. Both have now become a part of my daily routine as a result. Not only did Chris teach me to pay more attention to what I'm putting into my body, but he has shown me that healthy choices are far easier to make than I initially thought. As a result, it's now my habit to read all labels when buying groceries and I aim for more fresh than processed foods like I would have before. As a side result I discovered that I actually have a love of cooking! I now know that most of the cravings I had for the bad foods of before were a simple vitamin deficiency, I no longer have as intense cravings and am able to make a healthy substitute when they do come! I must be honest that I did miss some workouts and not eat great at every meal, I am only human after all, however, I am down by 22 lbs overall and still losing!! my ending weight after only 30 days is a staggering 219 lbs. Chris Walker has given me back control of myself while showing me that being healthy isn't difficult when you form new habits that work with you! Thank you so much Chris Walker for not only helping me to change my body and mindset but helping me shape my future!!

–Allan

Personal Support

I Would Love To Be Apart Of Your Life

I hope you've found this information valuable. I'm truly thankful for all that I've been through because now I understand how to help people like you, who may be struggling with an Overweight Mindset and an unsupportive Emotional Blueprint. I would love to connect with you further, to see if I can help you rewrite your Emotional Blueprint or whatever else you need help with so that you can reach your ideal weight more quickly, get healthy, and never put the weight back on!

To grab your free 30-minute Weight Loss and Health Consult with me, just go to the website address below. It will be fun because I'm cool and it's free! I promise!

www.coachwithchris.ca

Healthy Nutrition Lifestyle Accelerator

Hey Boss Ladies, Career Moms, and Students! I'm a Nutritionist, Weight Loss, and Mindset Coach that can help you to naturally control your weight without keto, strict dieting, or strenuous workouts!

After personally working with thousands of women who've struggled with their weight for years, and having completed over 150,000 client sessions we've successfully helped thousands of women end their struggle with weight gain, bad habits, hormonal, digestion, and emotional problems.

I'm also the only professional that's offering a 100 lb weight loss Guarantee. Let me help you master nutrition, eliminate bad habits and quickly make healthy lifestyle changes so you can naturally take control of your weight for the rest of your life!

Having lost both of my parents to illnesses that could have been prevented, I know just how important your health is!

As a result of this experience and my own weight challenges, I created the Healthy Nutrition Lifestyle Accelerator Program. Visit the website address below to learn more.

www.coachwithchris.ca

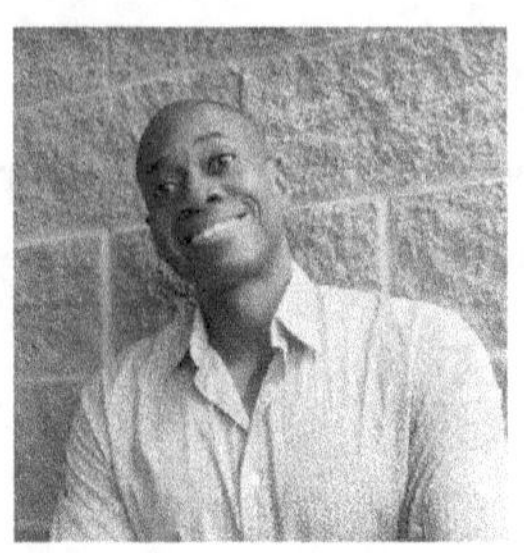

About the Author

Chris Walker is the founder of Coach With Chris, based out of Ontario Canada. He's a husband, father, and lover of everything natural! He specializes in helping professional women who struggle with weight loss to master nutrition, eliminate bad habits, and make healthy lifestyle changes so they can finally lose weight and keep it off.

Chris developed his passion for health after losing both of his parents to illnesses by the young age of 21. His father passed away from a stroke when he was 14, and then his mother succumbed to type 2 diabetes and colon cancer. Chris used these devastating losses to fuel his studies in health and start his coaching business that completed over 150, 000 client sessions.

Chris has helped women to get in shape for their wedding day as well as people battling severe obesity. Chris likes to focus on emotional health, habits, and mindset and only incorporates holistic methods and natural foods into his programs. Chris is a firm believer in a strong mind and guarantees results for those who don't mind a little hard work. Chris modestly likes to be referred to as a Nutritionist and Weight Loss Coach although he has many years of education from various institutions.

He is a Natural Nutrition Clinical Practitioner, (NNCP) Holistic Nutritionist, (HN) Functional Diagnostic Nutrition Practitioner, (FDN) Holistic Health Coach, Certified Personal Trainer and he's currently studying for his Doctorate and Ph.D. in Natural and Integrative Medicine. Chris is also a member of the Canadian Association of Natural Nutrition Professionals, (CANNP) and International Sports Sciences Association, (ISSA) Chris has made media appearances on Global Television, Rogers Daytime, and The Record News Paper and is a published author of many health and fitness-related articles and books.

You can connect with me on:

- https://coachwithchris.ca
- https://twitter.com/coachwchris
- https://www.facebook.com/coachwchris
- https://coachwithchris.ca/book-resources

Subscribe to my newsletter:

- https://coachwithchris.ca/free-offer